C^{THE}ommon Cold
C^{AND}ommon Sense

Other Books by Dale Alexander

Arthritis and Common Sense, 1950
Revised October 1951, September 1953

Good Health and Common Sense, 1960

*How I Stopped Growing Bald
and Started Growing Hair,* 1969

The Common Cold and Common Sense

How You Catch the Common Cold
and How You Can Avoid It

by Dale Alexander

NASH PUBLISHING • LOS ANGELES

Illustrations by Laurie Jordan

Excerpts in this book are reprinted
from *The Common Cold* by Christopher Andrewes.
By permission of W. W. Norton & Company, Inc.
Copyright © 1965 by Christopher Andrewes.

Library of Congress Catalog Card Number: 73-143000
Standard Book Number: 8402-1172-4

Published simultaneously in the United States and
Canada by Nash Publishing, 9255 Sunset Boulevard,
Los Angeles, California 90069.

Printed in the United States of America

First printing

I wish to express my appreciation
to Ethel Davis, my editor,
for her enormous help in the conception,
writing and completion of this work.

D. A.

Contents

Part III Vulnerability

Part IV Remedies

Part V Nutrition

List of Illustrations

Introduction

I have spent considerable time researching the common cold in medical literature at university and public libraries, with clinical investigators, virologists and common cold victims. The scientific consensus is that the major cold-causative virus is the rhinovirus strain. However, the record of the Common Cold Research Unit in Salisbury, England, acknowledges that ". . . there seem to be times when rhinoviruses are easy to isolate and other times when something else seems to be causing the prevalent colds, for nothing can be grown. An average figure would seem to lie somewhere near 25–30 percent for isolations of rhinoviruses. The number of infections is doubtless rather higher, perhaps 50 percent, since, as already indicated, a rhinovirus cannot always be recovered even from the colds which it has induced. There nevertheless remain large numbers of colds of which the cause is unknown. . . ."

I BELIEVE THAT I HAVE FOUND THE SOLUTION
TO THE MAJOR CAUSE OF THE COMMON COLD,
AND HAVE, THEREFORE, WRITTEN THIS BOOK TO
BRING MY FINDINGS TO THE PUBLIC.

I acknowledge with great respect and gratitude the work done by Sir Christopher Andrewes and his associates at the Common Cold Research Unit in Salisbury, England, as well as that done at the many research centers in the United States and other parts of the world. I have taken the results of their scientific experiments into consideration in the development of my theory. However, I found very little evidence of work done on the relationship of nutrition to the common cold; I, therefore, had to pioneer in this field.

Though I recognize that there are many circumstances under which one may possibly catch the common cold, no one to date has found the precise cause of the common cold. In this book I expose the *negative eating habits* which I found to be responsible for the common cold. I also present a *positive nutrition program,* which, if followed, will help build resistance against the common cold. Finally, the mystery of the common cold has been solved by me, and this solution is presented in this book.

It is my hope that the common cold researchers will study my work and then recognize the validity of my theories; further, that the layman will follow my suggestions, which will ensure him good health, free of the common cold.

I am at the moment
Deaf in the ears,
Hoarse in the throat,
Red in the nose,
Green in the gills,
Damp in the eyes,
Twitchy in the joints,
And fractious in temper
From a most intolerable
And oppressive cold.

—CHARLES DICKENS

Part I
New Discovery

1. The Origin of
My Theory

As a boy I was always robust, healthy and active. But three or four times a year a cold would strike me down. I could always tell I had one, because there would be a scratchy feeling in my throat, occasional chills, and my nose would start running.

My first thoughts were, oh no, this means three or four days of many handkerchiefs and bed rest. I would lie in bed and not move at all, hoping it would keep my nose from running. Each cold would last a few days to a week. Sometimes I would catch one cold on top of another. Occasionally I would run a point or two of fever.

I had a newspaper route all through my junior high and high school years, and I awoke to the alarm clock daily at 4:00 A.M. I trudged four to five miles each day, using shortcuts as I delivered my morning papers. It was two hours work.

During the winter, my feet became cold and wet as I delivered four hundred newspapers. The spring rains, and then the wet lawns in the summer, soaked my canvas sneakers and my trousers. Though I was exposed to the elements daily, the colds came only sporadically.

The common cold—what was its cause? It never occurred to me to search for an answer. I went on for years accepting colds as nuisances that everyone had every so often.

The First Clue

Some years later, my wife and I started a family in New York. We were blessed with a son. Four years later in Boston, our daughter was born. Both were healthy children.

When our son, Dean, was six and our daughter, Joan, was two, I worked as a medical technologist in Newington, Connecticut. We managed to save enough money to buy a second-hand Oldsmobile. We started taking occasional Sunday trips to Middletown, twelve miles from Newington, to visit my sister and her family.

I began to notice that after certain trips to my sister's, our son would wake up on Monday mornings with a cold. This caused me to wonder about these trips. What was happening? I had to look into this further.

I have always observed people. I have studied what they eat, how they eat and the condition of their skin and hair. I have looked for some indication of the relationship between food, eating habits and appearance.

Reviewing my son's colds, bearing in mind my concern with eating habits, I discovered that my sister would give my son a sweet every time we left for home. It was either a piece

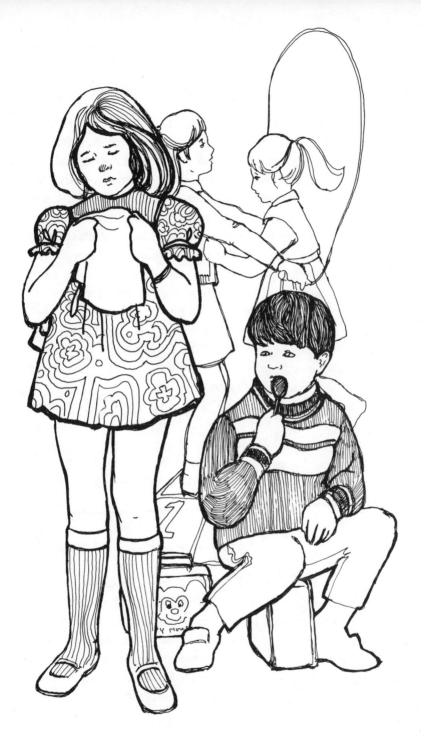

AFTER EATING THE STICKY SWEET, HIS COLD WAS BORN THE NEXT
DAY.

of chocolate, a lollypop, a chocolate cookie or a slice of chocolate cake. None was given to my daughter, who was content with her bottle of warm milk. At dinner we all ate the same food. My sister did not serve dessert. I realized the difference was that my son was the only one who ate a sweet, which he would save until he played with his friends at home.

One day the thought came through to me with great force: Someway, somehow, there was a relationship between my son's colds and the sweets he had eaten. He was the only one of us who ate a sweet on the Sundays we took the trips. *He was the only one who had a cold on the following Monday.*

Sometime after he ate the sweet, while playing with his friends, somehow his cold was born. I was excited by this clue of sweets. Though no one to whom I talked gave it any import, I felt I should research it.

At that time, in 1954, I knew nothing about common cold viruses. The family doctor told my wife, "Your son probably picked up a virus." What virus? Where did the virus come from? How did it get into our son? *Why was he the only one in the family affected by the virus after certain trips to my sister's?*

The Second Clue

At that time I chanced upon a book, *The Common Cold and How to Fight It,* by Dr. Noah Darrell Fabricant, published in 1945, which proved very stimulating. Dr. Fabricant states that "the normal nose gets a new mucous film about once every twenty minutes." He further states that a thin blanket of mucus lies directly on top of the cilia, which move this thin blanket of secretion toward the back part of the nose and throat. "As the mucus flows back toward the nasal pharynx, eventually to be discharged or swallowed, it is replaced by additional secretions from the glands in the mucous membrane."

I, therefore, deduced that if there is an irritant in the throat, this mucous film will sweep it out after twenty minutes.

The idea came to me that chocolate, or other sticky sweets, is the key *irritant,* and the *mechanism* in removing it is the movement of the new mucous film every twenty minutes.

The Third Clue

I read of the research done at the Common Cold Research Unit in Salisbury, England by Sir Christopher Andrewes, Dr. David A. J. Tyrrell, and others. Their work gave me another clue, the role of the viruses in the common cold.

I realized that there is some relationship between the mucous lining of the throat irritated by chocolate, or any sticky sweet, and common cold viruses. It was then that I felt compelled to explore my ideas further and develop my theory.

2. The Major Cause of the Common Cold

What is a cold? Briefly, the common cold is one of a number of virus infections which affect, often repeatedly, the lining of the nose, throat and other passages leading to the lungs.

It was of utmost importance in solving the mystery of the common cold to discover that chocolate and other sticky sweets irritate the mucous lining of the throat. If there is injury to the mucosa, this lowers the natural barrrier against infection. The balance is tipped. Therefore, when this irritation in the throat occurs, one is *immediately vulnerable* to the common cold.

To understand the problem of the common cold, it is vital to know what viruses are. I will, therefore, cite definitions from medical literature:

A virus is a minute infectious agent which, with certain exceptions, is not resolved by the light microscope, lacks independent metabolism and is able to replicate only within a living cell; the individual particle, or elementary body, consists of DNA or RNA, but not both, contained with a protein coat, which may be multi-layered.[1]

A virus consists essentially of a coil of a very complicated organic chemical, nucleic acid, which carries with it all the information, the specifications, necessary for making more virus of the same sort. . . . Associated with the nucleic acid is protein, a primary function of which seems to be to protect the precious nucleic acid from being destroyed by hostile mechanical substances in this environment. Another function is probably to make specific contact with the cell to be infected. . . . Viruses differ from bacteria in some ways of practical importance to laboratory workers. But they differ from bacteria not only in size, in their parasitic life within the cell and their resistance to drugs; it is now believed that they differ from all other living things in their mode of multiplication . . . .[2]

Viruses which are partly responsible for the common col fall into four categories:

(1) The Picorna Viruses
    Rhinoviruses
    Reoviruses
    Echo II
    Coxsackie A21

---

[1] *Dorland's Pocket Medical Dictionary* 21st ed. (Philadelphia: W. Saunders Co.). Used by permission.
[2] Sir Christopher Andrewes, *The Common Cold.*

(2) The Myxoviruses
   Para-influenza
   Influenza

(3) The Adenoviruses

(4) The Respiratory Synctial Virus

Rhinoviruses and Myxoviruses

The majority of research workers have concentrated on the rhinovirus strains as being the major common cold viruses. According to *Microbiology*, by Bernard D. Davis, M.D., *et al*, more than seventy-five strains of rhinoviruses have been isolated in England and the United States. It has been established that rhinoviruses cause rhinitis, but they can also infect the lower respiratory tract and cause pharyngitis. The rhinovirus adsorbs to a susceptible cell. It is taken inside the cell

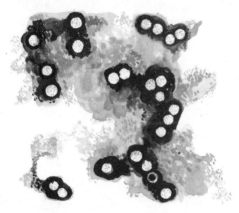

RHINOVIRUS—A MAJOR VIRUS, PARTLY RESPONSIBLE FOR THE COMMON COLD. MORE THAN SEVENTY-FIVE STRAINS ISOLATED IN THE UNITED STATES AND ENGLAND.

by a process called pinocytosis, where it is acted upon by cellular enzymes which free the nucleic acid from inside its protein coat. This nucleic acid has information which in effect programs the cell to replicate the virus. These viruses are replicated in the cytoplasm of the cell. The nucleic acid is RNA type.

I have followed the research work with rhinoviruses and appreciate the value of it in experimental work done with volunteers. However, after extensive study and thought, I have concluded that the *myxovirus strain should be given more attention in solving the problem of the common cold.* Myxoviruses are so-called because of their affinity for mucous (myxo) substances on the surfaces of the cells they infect. The myxovirus is surrounded by a lipoprotein envelope through which protrude an array of stubby protein spikes. These spikes cover the surface of the particle so it somewhat resembles a sea cucumber, and the tips of the spikes, which make contact with the cell surface prior to infection, are believed to contain an enzyme called neuraminidase. The myxovirus adsorbs to a susceptible cell. After digestion of the virus and release of the RNA, the RNA now goes to the nucleus of the cell where it is replicated. The RNA leaves the nucleus and is assembled into a completed viral particle at the cell membrane.

The Cilia, the Respiratory "Vacuum Cleaner"

Because the cilia are a strong defense against any infection of the respiratory tract, I shall deal with them at this point. Cilia are almost microscopic hairlike wands which cover the mucous membrane and which move back and forth like a field of wheat in a wind. They are as close together as the

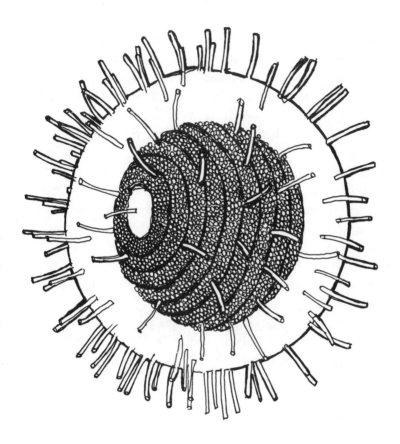

Myxovirus—a major virus, partly responsible for the common cold. The tips of the spikes make contact with cell surface prior to infection.

"hair" on a rug. They move secretions along the surface of the respiratory tract. By their rapid movement in waves, they propel bacteria or foreign particles, such as dust, toward the exterior of the body, whence, in normal circumstances, they are ejected. It has been established that the cilia move at the rate of about six hundred times a minute. Therefore, it can be readily seen that the cilia serve the respiratory tract as a "vacuum cleaner."

At this time I should like to call attention to the work of Dr. B. Hoorn and Dr. D. A. J. Tyrrell, as reported in the *British Journal of Experimental Pathology,* vol. 46, 1965. They demonstrated that representative strains of the common cold multiplied only in columnar ciliated cells as found in the human respiratory tract. Dr. B. Hoorn found that viruses can damage the epithelium to such an extent that ciliary activity ceases. This can be detected by microscopic examination. The person with repeated colds has the added problem of cilia replacement.

Further substantiation of virus replication was done by Dr. D. A. J. Tyrrell and his associate, Dr. M. L. Bynoe. They proved that common cold viruses can be readily cultivated in

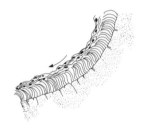

THE CILIA—RESPIRATORY TRACT "VACUUM CLEANER."

organ cultures of the nasal or tracheal epithelium of human embryos.

In a subsequent chapter, "The Important Role of Sound Nutrition," I will discuss cilia nourishment.

My Theory of What Causes Most Common Colds

How Chocolate and Other Sticky Sweets
Irritate the Throat Lining

Chocolate or other sticky sweets leave a residue which covers the throat lining for a period of about twenty minutes. Surrounding the mucous cells in the throat lining, there is a substance known as mucopolysaccharides, which is made up of protein and sugars. The sticky residue in the throat digests off the mucopolysaccharides. In other words, the residue causes an irritation in the throat lining, which in turn erodes the sugar-protein substance around the cell. *At this point there is injury to the mucosa—mucous membrane—*and the result is an approximate twenty-minute vulnerability to a virus. This physiological process is the first step in the development of most colds if the chocolate or other sticky sweet is eaten in the presence of someone with a cold who transmits the viable, common cold virus at the same time.

How the Common Cold Virus Attacks the Throat Lining

The irritated throat lining is a fertile area for the virus attack—the second step in the development of the cold. The

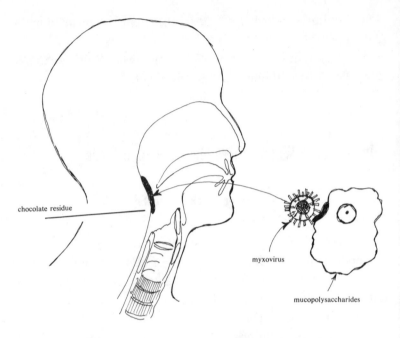

chocolate residue

myxovirus

mucopolysaccharides

THE RESIDUE FROM CHOCOLATE OR OTHER STICKY SWEETS IN THE
THROAT DIGESTS OFF THE MUCOPOLYSACCHARIDES.

virus now becomes attached to the mucous cell membrane
within the throat lining.

What occurs when this happens is set forth by Dr. John
Holland, of the University of Washington, as follows: "When
the virus becomes attached to the membrane, it appears to
'tickle' it. The membrane retreats a little, curling in and taking
the virus with it until a small depression forms beneath the
particle. It sinks deeper until the virus is sitting in a little
pouch or cover, surrounded on three sides by cell membrane.
Then cytoplasmic arms form a clasp around the particle. The

cell membrane surrounding the virus is pinched off and the Trojan horse is completely within the walls."[1]

Other scientists have pointed out that the tickling sensation prior to the cold is caused by electrostatic forces when viruses and cells are attracted to one another.

However, I should like to add my belief that when a person is infected with the virus he soon feels a "tickle" in the throat. This is a definite indication of the beginning of a cold. *This tickle comes about as a result of the spike-covered myxovirus'*

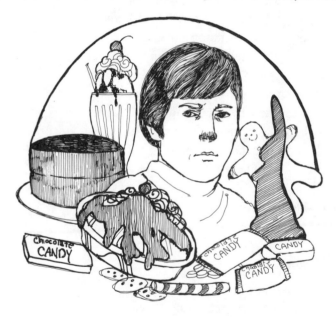

CAUSE OF MOST COLDS.

---

[1]Helena Curtis, *The Viruses,* © 1965 by Helena Curtis. Reprinted by permission of Doubleday & Company, Inc.

or other common cold virus' attack on the chocolate-sticky-sweet-irritated cells.

Synchronized Timing

As already stated, when a person eats chocolate or another sticky sweet in the presence of someone with a cold, he will in most cases catch cold. In connection with my original theory of what causes the common cold, the matter of synchronized timing is an essential factor. The length of time a person is vulnerable to the common cold, because he has eaten chocolate or another sticky sweet, is approximately twenty minutes, the time the sweet residue remains in the throat until the mucous film sweeps it out. Coincidentally, the virus which has been transmitted by a common cold carrier or by any other means becomes attached to the irritated cell. In order for a cold to develop, the virus must attack the mucous cell within the twenty minutes of vulnerability. In other words, *a cold will result if the virus-attack time is synchronized with the twenty-minute vulnerability time.*

The Result

Following infection by the virus, there is an incubation period which varies according to the virus—the third step in the development of the cold. The fourth step is a full-blown cold the following day.

The symptoms include all or part of the following: a sore throat, stuffed nose, sneezing, watery discharge, chest congestion, headache or sinus ache, cough, slight fever and a general feeling of discomfort.

Résumé of the Major Cause of the Common Cold

When someone eats a piece of chocolate or other sticky sweet, it causes an irritation of the mucous cell membrane of the throat lining. If a myxovirus or any common cold virus enters the throat (transmitted by someone present with a cold), it attaches to the irritated mucous cell membrane of the throat lining. The virus becomes imbedded in the mucous cells of the throat lining. If the virus-attack time is synchronized with the approximate twenty-minute vulnerability time, following a period of incubation, a full-blown cold results.

THE CHOCOLATE OR OTHER STICKY SWEET IS THE *CLUE* TO THE MYSTERY OF THE COMMON COLD. THE COMBINATION OF IRRITATION—INJURY—OF THE MUCOUS CELL MEMBRANE OF THE THROAT LINING FROM CHOCOLATE OR OTHER STICKY SWEET AND INFECTION FROM MYXOVIRUS OR ANY OTHER COMMON COLD VIRUS IS THE *MAJOR CAUSE OF THE COMMON COLD.*

3. The Harmful Effects of Chocolate and Other Sticky Sweets

Since chocolate and other sticky sweets make one vulnerable to the common cold, we must be aware that there are many different ways in which chocolate is prepared for consumption and avoid these confections.

It is important to note that manufacturers of chocolate candies also pour melted chocolate over other confections—to create a larger market for their sweets, in all forms. They also produce large variations of light or dark, sweet or bitter chocolate products. How many tons of nuts and raisins have been sold because of the addition of chocolate? So, in this age of sweets, sweets and more sweets, chocolate has become the most tempting, popular flavor and covering for almost every kind of confection.

I remember, as a youngster, attending hundreds of movies which I felt would not be complete unless I nibbled on a

Baby Ruth or an Oh Henry bar. And when I grew bored with them, there were all the other endless varieties and combinations of chocolate to munch on. I had no inkling at that time of the danger of chocolate and did not relate my occasional colds to it.

To this day I suspect that my older sister's migraine headaches were due to her eating large quantities of chocolate kisses in her youth. And, I can recognize the unquestionable damage that eating many boxes of chocolate did to my wife's body. Over a period of fourteen years, she had had thirteen skin grafts on her leg which had been seriously burned by fire at the age of six months. Each time she had surgery, scores of people would visit her in the Massachusetts General Hospital and bring her boxes of chocolates. By the time she was fifteen years of age, she had gained about fifty pounds, as she ate box after box of chocolates. As surely as one is addicted to cigarets, she was hooked on chocolate.

How vividly I remember the first year of our married life, in which she was critically ill in a New York hospital with streptococcal sore throat. Thereafter, in the following years, she had a number of recurrences.

The only luxury we could afford in our early years of marriage was one or two movies a week in the neighborhood theatre. She would never pass the candy counter in the lobby of the theatre without buying a candy bar. Whenever we entertained in our home, she would immediately be prompted to purchase boxes of chocolates. Two other of her favorite candies were clusters of chocolate-covered raisins and nuts. Neither of us was aware at the time that the candy manufacturers had certainly done a job of adulterating the nutritious nut and raisin. Because I had a weight problem, I refrained from eating sweets.

Now, years later, as a result of my research which led to the solution of what causes the common cold, how clearly the pieces seem to fit together: her hospitalization, the lobby of the theatre, the chocolate bar—the throat irritant—the crowded theatre with sniffling people, virus prevalence, virus incubation during that night and the next day or two, culminating in the inevitable cold, sore throat and occasional streptococcal infection.

Beyond our own immediate family, I am aghast at the millions who eat quantities of candies, cookies, cakes and combinations of sweets that are flavored or decorated with the harmful chocolate.

Milk and the Addition of Chocolate

In the past, the people of this country were content with wholesome, health-bearing milk. But now, in the twentieth century, chocolate milk has been made available and is sold in enormous quantities to those who favor it to ordinary milk. How many hundreds of thousands of children, yes, even millions, have had chocolate milk placed in front of them as a tasty substitute for milk. There are those who think that chocolate milk is just milk with chocolate added, but this is not so. Tons of white sugar are poured into the chocolate milk mixture to provide the sweetness people like, and which leads to the tremendous sale of this harmful beverage. In addition to causing common cold vulnerability, the chocolate and white sugar content create an imbalancing effect on the calcium and phosphorus levels in the bloodstream.

Because of constant consumption of chocolate milk, many youngsters' digestive systems are damaged, resulting in constipation. Later, as chronic constipation persists, there is the inevitable painful condition known as hemorrhoids.

How I wish the manufacture of chocolate milk could be outlawed. This would prevent children's habitual consumption of chocolate, which is so injurious. Yet I know this would be futile, because the chocolate manufacturers have seen to it that mothers, with the aid of chocolate syrup, can make their own chocolate milk. It is distressing to realize that countless children, therefore, are definitely enslaved by cold-causing chocolate milk.

Between commercially made chocolate milk and chocolate milk mixed in the home, the one made at home is more harmful. Visualize a glass of milk and at the bottom a tablespoon of thick, chocolate syrup which has not been thoroughly mixed into the milk. When the child swallows this sticky chocolate syrup, his throat lining becomes coated with this irritant, which can lead to a cold. The commercially made chocolate leaves less residue to irritate the throat, because it is homogenized. However, because it contains chocolate, it nevertheless is harmful.

The craze for chocolate persists among teenagers in the form of chocolate milkshakes, which are also injurious. Think of the danger and damage that the combination of chocolate milkshakes, hamburgers and French fries have on the skin of young people. The combination of the iced chocolate drink and the hot oil in the fried food makes it almost impossible to assimilate the oil properly. As a consequence, there is harm to the skin and the body. In particular, the shafts leading from the sebaceous glands become plugged. This, in my opinion, can start an acne condition.

EVERY CHOCOLATE-MILK DRINKER IS A POTENTIAL COLD VICTIM!

Chocolate Candy

I would say that children between the ages of four and sixteen are the biggest buyers of chocolate candy. It is, therefore, logical and obvious to me, after considerable thought and research, that chocolate candy is one of the reasons why children catch more colds than adults.

Perhaps the greatest chocolate-decorated foods are the nut and the raisin. This combination, with some sort of filler, is put together with either sugar, sucrose or a sweetening extract and then molded into a candy bar. There are many hundreds of other kinds of manufactured candy bars in the United States. There is a chocolate candy bar called "Chunky," with actually only one bite to it. As small as it is, it too is filled with the favored nut and raisin combination. There is a candy made of peanut butter covered by melted chocolate, which is another favorite. An often-consumed sweet is the bitter yet pleasant-tasting candy mint, which is bitter chocolate poured over a minted center. And there is home-made fudge, an all-time choice.

In every country of the world, the candy bar can be found in the candy store, drug store, little shop, railroad station, airport, department store and supermarket, at sports events, newspaper counters, theatres, on the streets—literally everywhere. Because of this, in my extensive travels throughout the world on lecture tours, I have made every effort to warn the audiences that every variation of chocolate is harmful.

EVERY CHOCOLATE-CANDY EATER IS A POTENTIAL COLD VICTIM!

Lollypops

An unfortunate mistake that many a mother makes is to use the lollypop as an inducement for the child to eat his meat and vegetables. She tempts her child with lollypops in every color and flavor. What child can resist this delicacy! Lollypops are, in many cases, a daily "treat" in the mother-child reward relationship and therefore constitutes a daily common cold threat. The sweet, sticky substance in the lollypop adheres to the throat lining and irritates it, making the lollypop eater highly vulnerable to the common cold if there is someone present with a cold. For visual proof, observe the expectoration from ten to twenty minutes after the lollypop is consumed. It will contain the colored, sticky evidence which is the throat lining irritant.

EVERY LOLLYPOP EATER IS A POTENTIAL COLD VICTIM!

Ice Cream with Chocolate

Our great-grandmothers and grandmothers made ice cream at home. They used natural, sweet cream and natural sweetening agents. This was a healthful sweet, as it did not contain any throat-irritating ingredients. However, within the last fifty years or so, the chocolate-covered ice cream popsicle and sandwich have become available. Unfortunately for health's sake, they are consumed frequently in exorbitant quantities by people of all ages.

I recommend careful judgment when selecting ice cream. Ice cream should not be eaten when under a layer of chocolate. Ice cream should not be eaten when under a sprinkling of chocolate jimmies. Ice cream should not be eaten when under melted chocolate fudge. Ice cream should not be eaten with any sticky, sweet sauce. ICE CREAM SHOULD BE EATEN PLAIN OR WITH SIMPLE FRESH FRUIT.

EVERY CHOCOLATE-COVERED ICE CREAM EATER IS A POTENTIAL COLD VICTIM!

Cakes

Like candy, cake is made in many eye-appealing variations. The most irresistible of all is the chocolate-frosted cake. It is, many say, the most delicious. However, it too should be avoided, as it irritates the throat lining. I cannot emphasize enough that chocolate must not be eaten in any form if there is anyone present with the common cold.

Sticky frostings such as butterscotch, mocha or even plain white are just as dangerous as chocolate because they also irritate the throat lining. A warning! Regardless of what type of frosted cake you plan to serve, if there is anyone in the room with the common cold, I suggest that you put the cake in the freezer.

One particularly encouraging point! Any kind of cake may be eaten if there is no one present with the common cold. However, one must, at the same time, be aware that sugar lowers resistance to the common cold. If you are a cake lover and can't do without it, there are some without frostings which are safe to eat. Three that come to mind are cheese cake, sponge cake and pound cake.

EVERY CHOCOLATE- AND STICKY-FROSTED-CAKE EATER IS A POTENTIAL COLD VICTIM!

Cookies and Pies

In many families there are those who do not care for cake or pie. They much prefer cookies, especially for TV snacks. As a consequence, ours has become a nation of cookie eaters. If anyone questions this, just look at the tremendous sections of cookies on display in the supermarkets.

Most cookies contain the ever present chocolate. One in particular is the brownie, which is generally covered with chocolate fudge. We now know that such sweets have an abrasive effect on the throat lining.

The housewife who prefers to make her own cookies usually favors the Toll House cookie. Here again, pieces of chocolate are blended into the batter. It is regrettable that chocolate is a part of just about every sweet.

EVERY CHOCOLATE-COOKIE EATER IS A POTENTIAL COLD VICTIM!

Fortunately, not all people eat large quantities of chocolate daily. The reasons for abstinence are fear of the resultant stomach ache, the realization that it can cause cavities in teeth, the gaining of weight and migraine headaches.

Further Dangers

Apart from the fact that chocolate in any form can be cold-causing, it should be avoided because:

(1) It has *no* natural sweetening. Therefore, it is sweetened with refined white sugar, which lowers resistance to the common cold, or with artificial sweeteners, which impair the vitamin B content stored in the body.

(2) Chocolate contains theobromine which is a stimulant similar to the harmful caffeine in coffee.

(3) Chocolate contains oxalic acid. When chocolate is used in milk, the oxalic acid prevents the calcium and phosphorus from being properly assimilated. Since milk is the major source of calcium, which is needed in children to build good bones and teeth, it must not be contaminated with chocolate.

(4) Oxalic acid and theobromine, found in chocolate, are low-level, toxic elements to which many people are allergic.

(5) Surveys show that conservatively 20 percent to 25 percent of all age groups cannot eat chocolate without adverse reaction. For example, most older people who eat chocolate, suffer from liver impairment, nausea and headaches. Teenagers who eat excessive amounts of chocolate are usually plagued with varying degrees of skin acne.

In conclusion, below is an excellent and important article

which appeared in the *Los Angeles Times,* November 26, 1954, under the title "Chocolate Can Be Dangerous":

New York—Chocolate, the opiate of the sneaker set, triggers allergic reactions that may be severe or bizarre in many more children than is generally realized, a Brooklyn physician warns.

Dr. Joseph H. Fries said these "sleeper reactions" may range in seriousness from skin rashes to vomiting and can mimic other ailments such as measles and hay fever.

"Chocolate consumption in this country is enormous," he told the American Academy of Pediatrics national meeting here. "It is cleverly blended as an additive or flavoring in a variety of goods such as milks, candies and cakes.

"But it precipitates allergic reactions more often than chocolate manufacturers are willing to admit," Dr. Fries added.

The allergy director at Methodist Hospital said he had tested 300 children afflicted with a variety of allergies and found that 200 were sensitive to chocolate, including 25 who had severe reactions.

Complicating the problem, Dr. Fries said, is the fact that "chocolate ingestion may become a habit of a child like smoking and drinking by his parents because it gives psychological gratification and releases tensions.

"In other words, chocolate may be to the child what cigarets are to the adult," Dr. Fries said.

He added that trying to keep chocolate from an allergic child "has psychological overtones similar to those met by an adult who is trying to stop smoking." He said withdrawal is even more difficult if the child's mother has given him chocolate or chocolate milk as a reward or a pacifier.

Fortunately, Dr. Fries said, allergies to chocolate and other foods such as milk, eggs, fish, nuts, oranges and beans tend to diminish as the child gets older.

He added that St. John's bread, a chocolate substitute made from the fruit of the carob tree, which "tastes, smells, looks and defies detection from the original," is available to parents having children who are not only allergic to chocolate but also hooked on it.

Nowhere in literature have I seen anything that relates chocolate to the common cold. I do so! This book presents my theory that chocolate can trigger the common cold.

Part II
Research and
Experimental Proof

4. Résumé of Historical Research into the Common Cold

The common cold has been an enigma for centuries. Though extensive work has been done, the medical profession has failed to find the cause of the common cold. It was when viruses were isolated and labeled in the laboratory that significant headway was achieved.

Within this chapter, I will give a chronological résumé of experimental findings by medical researchers. Their work proved invaluable to me in the development of my theory.

Experimental Findings in 1914

Dr. Von W. Kruse demonstrated that the transmission of the nasal secretions from a person ill with a common cold could produce colds in previously well volunteers. These secretions were filtered through a Berkefeld filter before inoculation into the volunteers.[1]

Experimental Findings in 1930

Dr. A. R. Dochez and his associates studied the human respiratory tract during colds and concluded that the bacteria they found really belonged to the normal flora, but he and his aides successfully transmitted human and ape colds to chimpanzees by means of filtrates made from nasal secretion. Finally, after keeping their volunteers in strict isolation, they produced colds in man with filtrates from four of nine washings.[2]

Experimental Findings in 1933

A significant contribution was made by Dr. W. Smith and his co-workers when they cultivated the influenza type A in the further exploration of the viral respiratory diseases. This advancement opened the way for numerous investigations, including inoculation of attenuated strains into the volunteers. This was a forerunner to the development of a vaccine for epidemic influenza.[3]

---

[1]"Die Erreger von Husten und Schnupfen," *Münch Med. Wachensche* 61:1547 (1914).

[2]"Studies in the Common Cold. IV. Experimental Transmission of the Common Cold to Anthropoid Apes and Human Beings by Means of a Filterable Agent," *J. Exp. Med.* 52:701, (1930).

[3]"A Virus Obtained from Influenza Patients," *Lancet* 2:66 (1933).

Experimental Findings in 1934

Dr. W. F. Wells' study of airborne droplets and particles and their relationship in the transmission of the common cold was made in 1934. He found that soon after being formed, the larger droplets fall rapidly to the floor. The small droplets fall slowly and, because of their relatively large surface area, evaporate so rapidly that they are reduced to small, dry droplet nuclei before they reach the ground. These nuclei remain airborne indefinitely and can be carried long distances by air currents. It is quite often thought that infection is transmitted by this means in the case of colds, but there is in fact little evidence to support this view. Although such particles are formed and inhaled, many respiratory viruses lose their infectivity when dried in air. Airborne viruses have been detected more in large-sized droplet particles which fall to the ground than in airborne particles which are likely to be inhaled.[1]

Experimental Findings in 1941

Dr. R. B. Bourndillon's and his associates' study, using ultra-high-speed photographs taken of persons talking, showed that large numbers of airborne particles are produced from the mouth.[2]

Experimental Findings in 1946

Dr. J. P. Duguid found that many more particles are produced after a sneeze than when talking, but most of these are

---

[1]*Amer. J. Hyg.* 20:611 (1934).
[2]*Lancet* 2:365 (1941).

from the mouth and not from the nose. A cough produces a small number of particles which, again, come through the mouth, but in this case most of the particles are formed not from the saliva, but from respiratory secretions torn away from the mucous membranes of the lower respiratory tract.[1]

Experimental Findings in 1952

Dr. J. E. Lovelock's and associates' study established that the placing of infective secretions around the outside of the nose is unlikely to produce a cold. *A most unexpected finding was that the use of a contaminated handkerchief for twenty-four hours was quite inefficient for the purpose of passing the infection to a normal person.* These results are probably due to the sensitivity of virus to drying.[2]

Experimental Findings in 1955

Dr. H. S. Ginsberg's and associates' studies in military recruits in World War II were particularly productive of knowledge concerning nonbacterial diseases. Acute respiratory disease characterized by tracheitis, bronchitis, cough, sore throat and hoarseness was described and found to be caused by adenovirus 4.[3]

---

[1]*Brit. Med. J.* i. i:1453 (1946).

[2]*Lancet* 2:657 (1952).

[3]"Etiologie Relationship of the RI-67 Agent to Acute Respiratory Disease (ARD)," *J. Clin. Invest.* 34:820 (1955).

Experimental Findings in 1960

Dr. R. Parsons' and associates' study, using Coxsackie A21 virus, showed that infective secretions in the form of drops, caused only a mild upper respiratory infection, whereas fine aerosol (even in small doses) gave rise to marked lower respiratory symptoms accompanied by rhonchi and rales, which almost never occur with colds. This seems to indicate that viruses borne on large particles were more likely to be retained in the nose, whereas those carried in small particles reached the lower respiratory tract to produce lower respiratory infections. In general, children were found to be much more effective as spreaders of infection than adults, possibly because they cough and sneeze uninhibitedly and at distances close to their contacts.[1]

Experimental Findings in 1962

Dr. F. E. Buckland's and associates' study found that by using Coxsackie A21 virus to produce experimental colds it could be demonstrated that the maximum amounts of virus are in the nasal secretion and much less in the saliva or pharyngeal secretions. During normal talking or quiet respiration, almost no nasal material is expelled. In an inhibited or unsuccessfully smothered sneeze, virus is shed as nasal secretion, but even then, only about 0.01 or 0.1 cc is expelled, or only about 1 percent of this tiny amount is in a form which can stay airborne for only a minute or two. The majority of material is sneezed out in the form of large droplets which fall

---

[1] *Brit. Med. J.* i:1766 (1960).

quickly to the ground. As soon as virus-bearing particles are formed, the infectivity of the virus within them begins to drop. In general, the rhinoviruses survive better in cold, moist air than in warm, dry air.[1]

Experimental Findings in 1959 and 1963

Dr. George Gee Jackson's and associates' study at the University of Illinois contained serologic and clinical data which were presented to demonstrate two phenomena regarding the nature of respiratory disease viruses as they occur in human nasal secretions: (1) More than a single infectious agent may be present in nasal secretions during a natural cold; and (2) the disease-producing capacity of a respiratory virus may be appreciably altered by its passage in an alternative host.[2]

Experimental Findings in 1963

Dr. V. Knight's and associates' study at the Clinical Center of the National Institute of Health at Bethesda, Maryland, was similar to the work done by Andrewes in Salisbury, England, and by Jackson at the University of Illinois, where over one hundred viral agents were studied, and valuable informa-

---

[1]*Nature* 195:1063 (1962).

[2]"Transmission of the Common Cold to Volunteers under Controlled Conditions: IV. Specific Immunity to the Common Cold," *J. Clin. Invest.* 38:762 (1959). "Contributions of Volunteers to Studies on the Common Cold," Conference on Newer Respiratory Disease Viruses, *Amer. Rev. Resp. Dis.* 88 (Suppl.): 120 (1963).

tion about the role of these viruses in human respiratory disease was gathered by their combined efforts. The major part of these studies involved the characterization of the disease produced by newly isolated viruses. Other investigations have yielded information on the protective effect of serum and nasal antibody, and factors of resistance other than serum antibody have been examined. More recently volunteer studies have provided information on the effectiveness of respiratory virus vaccines.[1]

Experimental Findings in 1965

Dr. D. A. J. Tyrrell's study evaluated that infections with known viruses cannot account for all colds. In one experiment, the nasal secretions of a number of subjects with colds were examined for both bacteria and virus, but neither could be found, and yet these secretions produced colds when given to volunteers. The evidence seems to indicate the presence of a filterable virus which was not identifiable at that time.[2]

Experimental Findings in 1946-1966

Sir Christopher Andrewes' and associates' study at the Common Cold Research Unit, Salisbury, England, produced the greatest contribution towards new knowledge on the com-

---

[1]"Studies in Volunteers with Respiratory Viral Agents; Small Particle Aerosol; Heterotypic Protection; Viral Chemotherapy; Bovine Reovirus in Man," *Amer. Rev. Resp. Dis.* 88 (Supp.): 135 (1963).

[2]*Common Colds and Related Diseases* (London: Edward Arnold, Ltd., 1965).

mon cold. (See Chapter 5.) When serious work on this disease was started there in 1946, all that was known about the common cold was that it could be transmitted to human volunteers through experiments performed on volunteers.[1]

In the foregoing valuable experimental findings, the reader will note that no work was done in the field of nutrition and its relationship to the common cold. This vitally important area of study merited and demanded attention. I, therefore, spent many years toward that end. Now, finally, my findings are presented through this book.

---

[1]*Scientific American* 189:39 (1951).

5. The Common Cold Research Unit at Salisbury, England

It is important in viewing the work done in researching the common cold to turn to England. Starting in 1946, Sir Christopher Andrewes and other noted scientists spent over twenty years at the Common Cold Research Unit, Harvard Hospital, Salisbury, Wiltshire, England, trying to establish the cause and cure for the common cold. Their experiments created vast amounts of scientific knowledge on the common cold. However, they do not profess to have found the cause.

I have read Dr. Andrewes' report entitled "The Common Cold"[1] and have found that their efforts yielded significant results. I have also read Dr. Andrewes' book, *The Common*

---

[1]*Proceedings of the Royal Society of Medicine* 59 (July 1966).

Cold, which I found contained invaluable material. I have quoted from it throughout this book, as I believe it to be the most important work on the subject.

I am pleased to find in Dr. Andrewes' book, a chapter devoted to the Common Cold Research Unit at Salisbury. I shall quote from this to give a precise report:

> By 1946, some fifteen years had passed since Dochez's work on colds and nothing much had been done about it in the meantime. There had, however, in the intervening years been considerable gains in knowledge about viruses, very many of them having been cultivated in fertile developing hens' eggs.
>
> Some of us working at the National Institute for Medical Research (then at Hampstead, now at Mill Hill), accordingly laid plans for a fresh attack on the common cold, and the Medical Research Council agreed to support the enterprise. Knowledge about other viruses had been gained mainly by observing their effects on experimental animals, and more recently by cultivation in eggs. We had, however, no evidence that such techniques were available for colds. Chimpanzees, the only known susceptible animal, were far too expensive and difficult to handle. We had, therefore, to plan to use volunteers. Production of a cold in an inoculated volunteer was our only test for presence of cold virus. As a method of work it was horribly clumsy, expensive and unreliable, but it was all we had. Our first objective, therefore, would be to use this clumsy technique as a means of finding a better one, a laboratory test for presence of virus.

. . . Harvard Hospital at Salisbury turned out to be almost exactly what we wanted. . . . Volunteers were first obtained from university students on vacation. . . . To keep up the supply of volunteers, we have held annual press conferences, either in Salisbury or London, usually at the New Year when we most need to stimulate recruitment. . . .

. . . Volunteers . . . received a physical examination to ensure, as far as possible, that no one was already in the incubation stages of a naturally contracted cold. . . .

. . . At the end of the quarantine period a decision was reached as to suitability of each "guinea pig" for experiment. . . . Then the virologist came along with his materials for test. These consisted either of cold-filtrates expected to give some colds or of harmless "control" fluids or of material of unknown activity. . . .

. . . Materials under test were, in most trials, run up the nostrils of the subjects while they lay on their backs, heads tilted back. Neither volunteers nor clinical observer knew the nature of the inoculum. The doctor had to record in writing at the end of each trial which people in his opinion had colds; only then was he permitted to see the key to the code and to know what it all meant. Why was all this necessary? For this reason: it is easy to know if you have a streaming cold or no cold at all. But symptoms may be of almost every grade between these extremes. . . .

In deciding between "cold" or "no cold" the doctor finds the most useful criterion to be the amount of nasal secretion, as judged by the numbers of paper handkerchiefs used in a day. . . .

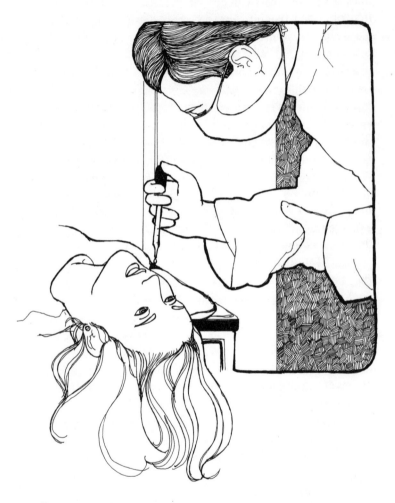

Fluid inserted in volunteer to test for the presence of virus.

Throat and nose are of course examined daily and often give positive evidence of presence of a cold; but on the whole the information they yield is slight compared with evidence of abnormal nasal secretion on the handkerchiefs. . . .

Results of work carried out at the Salisbury Unit from 1946 till about 1960 are difficult to interpret. We know now that very many colds are due to rhinoviruses, which have definite properties, but that some colds are caused by viruses belonging to different families and having quite other properties. Since, however, more naturally occurring colds in adults are caused by rhinoviruses than by other known agents, it is likely that a great many at least of our earlier findings did in fact concern rhinoviruses.

We had, of course, for our studies, no large supply of any one virus and we must have worked from time to time with several different ones. All the infective agents survived well when kept frozen at $-76°$ C the temperature of dry ice, and that was a help. Many germs survive better at $-76°$ C than when only just frozen. We inoculated a number of volunteers with a particular nose washing and made a big pool of the nose washings of all those who developed colds, trusting that the same agent was causing the colds in all of them. We did this on several occasions using different starting materials. We also obtained, and pooled, washings from a number of boys who were victims of an epidemic of colds at a big public school. These valuable pools were stored in our dry ice refrigerator.

. . . The symptoms produced by our washings [showed]

the various viruses did not behave alike. We obtained a varying number of "takes" in several years of research, at best 50 percent or a little higher, at worst only 28 percent. At first we thought that women were more susceptible than men but later the slight differences were evened out. Within our eighteen to forty or fifty age limits incidence was unaffected by age; nor was it influenced by time since the last recorded cold nor by history of tonsillectomy.

Clearly, if 50 percent or more of your experimental animals are going to be naturally resistant, it is necessary to test a number before a negative answer can be taken at its face value, since you may by chance strike a number of insusceptibles. So we usually tested six or eight people at least with any one material.

Our first efforts were directed to an attempt to cultivate a virus in fertile developing hens' eggs. Such methods had lately been applied with success to one virus after another. Four methods were available. Some viruses would grow on the delicate membranes surrounding the whole embryo, some when inoculated into the egg-yolk, some in amniotic fluid, . . . some in the larger volume of fluid, the allantoic fluid, into which the embryo's waste products are discharged. A great deal had been learnt about influenza viruses by these methods of cultivation and our hopes were high. Several hundreds of eggs were used. Attempted cultures by the four methods mentioned above were tested on twenty-eight, sixty-five, fifty-four and ninety-nine volunteers respectively. At first we were hopeful of success, but later found that some colds seemed to start up after we had given "control" uninoculated egg fluids, but this only happened erratically. One way and another, we finally decided that our viruses had probably not multiplied in eggs.

At about the same time workers in three different laboratories abroad claimed success in growing cold virus in eggs. They were kind enough to send us their material and we devoted much effort, especially in the most promising case, to an attempt to repeat the work. We unfortunately failed to do so. Reasons for discrepancies in the results are not clear. At the present time no laboratory, so far as I am aware, has under study a virus causing typical colds, cultivable in eggs.

Our next attempt was to find a susceptible laboratory animal rather less expensive and more readily available than the chimpanzee. We inoculated by various routes, but mainly by means of drops up the nose, mice, rats, guinea pigs, cotton-rats, voles, hamsters, grey squirrels, hedgehogs, ferrets, pigs, chicks and several species of monkey—green monkey, red patas, baboon and sooty mangabey. From several of these we tried to recover viruses with which to infect human beings, all in vain. A number of people told us that certain species were very apt to catch colds by contact with man: cats, capuchin monkeys and flying squirrels were particularly mentioned. But these proved no more susceptible to human cold viruses than the others we had tested. One of the South American capuchin monkeys is often called the Weeper because its eyes seem to be brimming over with tears and this fact may have deceived observers. Cats certainly get very bad colds and these are due to several different agents including, possibly, rhinoviruses—but cat rhinoviruses, not human ones.

We thus failed in our earlier attempts at finding the

laboratory technique for studying colds. While we continued the search it seemed well worth while to find out
what we could about the properties of our virus. We
could produce colds at times with material diluted
1:1000 but not more. The virus we tested was readily
inactivated by heating to 56° C. It survived, as already
mentioned, at −76° C and for at least two years. It was
apparently smaller than the influenza virus and passed a
filter with pores only 60 mµ across; so its diameter was
probably 30 mµ or less, that is three hundred thousandths
of a millimetre or about a millionth of an inch. A useful
tool in the attempt to classify viruses into families is to
see whether ether destroys their activity. We were puz-
zled because some of our tests indicated that ether did
destroy cold virus, while others gave an opposite result.
We can guess now that we were probably using rhinovirus (which is resistant to ether) in some experiments
and a different agent in others. On the whole, the most
useful results of our early studies at Salisbury concerned
attempts to find out something about the transmission of
colds from one person to another. . . .

In my search to solve the problem of the common cold I
have concentrated on the nutritional approach, which I am
convinced is instrumental in determining whether or not one
becomes a victim of the common cold.

In the literature regarding the experiments with volunteers
at the Common Cold Research Unit there was no mention of
the diet for the volunteers. I, therefore, wrote to Dr. Andrewes
requesting this information. Dr. D. A. J. Tyrrell, an associate
of Dr. Andrewes', was kind enough to answer: "The volun-

teers here receive a diet which is most simply described as normal home cooking and I enclose a sample menu. No television is provided and they are allowed half a pint of milk each day and one pint of beer, cyder or squash."

I have analyzed their menu. There are a few sticky sweets such as marmalade, iced buns, jam tarts and possibly Madeira cake. Since I do not know the circumstances under which the meals were eaten, I cannot determine to what extent these sweets contributed to any colds the volunteers contracted. However, I feel safe in speculating that if the sweets were eaten by one not infected with a cold, in the presence of a fellow volunteer who had contracted a cold, he would in all likelihood develop a cold.

I trust future experimentation with volunteers who are inoculated will take into consideration my theory that chocolate and other sticky sweets are cold-causing irritants. I am confident the results will be most rewarding.

The menu of Harvard Hospital is presented on the following pages.

Common Cold Research Unit—Harvard Hospital

	MONDAY	TUESDAY	WEDNESDAY
BREAKFAST	Cereal or Porridge Boiled Eggs Toast and Marmalade	Cereal or Porridge Bacon and Fried Bread Toast and Marmalade	Cereal or Porridge Bacon and Fried Bread Toast and Marmalade
BREAK	Coffee	Coffee	Coffee
LUNCH	Mince and Rice Peas Curry Sauce Baked Custard	Veal Patty Potatoes Carrots Fruit and Custard	Roast Beef Yorkshire Pudding Roast Potatoes Greens Baked Rice Pudding
TEA	Biscuits	Scones	Victoria Sponge
SUPPER	Fish Fingers Chips Biscuits and Cheese	Soup Scrambled Eggs Fresh Fruit	Macaroni and Cheese Jam Tarts

Bill of Fare for the Week

THURSDAY	FRIDAY	SATURDAY	SUNDAY
Cereal or Porridge	Cereal or Porridge	Cereal or Porridge	Cereal or Porridge
Haddock Fillets	Bacon and Tomatoes	Boiled Eggs	Bacon and Fried Bread
Toast and Marmalade	Toast and Marmalade	Toast and Marmalade	Toast and Marmalade
Coffee	Coffee	Coffee	Coffee
Irish Stew	Fried Fish	Stewed Steak	Roast Lamb
Potatoes	and Chips	and	Mint Sauce
Milk Jelly	Marmalade	Dumplings	Roast
	Pudding	Potatoes	Potatoes
		Carrots	Greens
		Banana	Fruit Pies
		Custard	
Iced Buns	Gingerbread	Madeira Cake	Madeira Cake
Shepherd's Pie	Sausages	Luncheon	Cold Ham
Biscuits and	Baked Beans	Meat	Cress
Cheese	Stewed Prunes	Crisps	Biscuits and
		Pickles	Cheese
		Biscuits and	Fresh Fruit
		Cheese	
		Fruit	

6. Further International Research with Volunteers

It is understandable that since nine thousand volunteers were tested in England for their susceptibility to catch the common cold, subsequent medical investigators in other parts of the world would find it necessary to use large numbers of people. In the United States, one research program at the University of Illinois, College of Medicine, Chicago, Illinois, conducted by Dr. George Gee Jackson, consisted of some four thousand volunteers who participated in a controlled study on the common cold over a period of nine years. In the course of Dr. Vernon Knight's investigation in Bethesda, Maryland, under the auspices of the Laboratory of Clinical Investigations and Laboratory of Infectious Diseases, four hundred volunteers participated over a period of two and a half years in a study of approximately twenty viral infections

75

other than the common cold. All three projects were working toward the same goal—the common cold.

Additional information on the Common Cold Research Unit's work has been reported by Dr. D. A. J. Tyrrell in "The Use of Volunteers.[1] Because this amplifies the material in the preceding chapter, I shall quote it herewith:

EXPERIMENTAL PROCEDURE USED AT THE COMMON COLD
RESEARCH UNIT, SALISBURY, ENGLAND

(1) The volunteers are allocated at random to experimental and control groups. Therefore, no one can presume that those living in a particular hut or those with particular initials are more likely to be given one material than the other.

(2) Volunteers are subdivided into small groups. As a result, when one volunteer develops a cold, only one or two others will be likely to receive the suggestion that they are likely to develop colds. As the subgroups have no contact with each other, it is also possible to work with several infectious agents in one trial.

(3) Volunteers given noninfectious materials are included in *every* experiment, so that there is a constant check on what might be called the "sensitivity" of the clinician and the subject. The control drops given match in color and taste those containing virus, and volunteers who receive them are given exactly the same instructions as those given infectious material. Over the year 1 or 2 percent of these control subjects are recorded as having colds; these may be errors of diagnosis or genuine infections, as will be discussed later.

---

[1]*American Review of Respiratory Diseases* 88 (September 1963).

(4) The inoculum is given by a laboratory worker who usually has no further contact with the volunteer. Thus, he cannot influence the results either deliberately or accidentally. He is the only person who knows what the volunteers have been given, and this information is passed to the clinical observer only after the latter has written down his opinion of the symptoms and signs observed in each volunteer.

Premature "leaking" of such information may affect the results in various ways. If the volunteer and observer are very enthusiastic, they will tend to overemphasize symptoms in those given virus and minimize those in controls. In other cases the observer may "lean over backwards" in order to avoid this sort of error and, in fact, bias his results in the opposite direction. The only way to avoid bias is to make it impossible, by keeping the observer and the observed completely ignorant of extraneous information which could influence their judgment. We encounter some difficulties in preserving this state of ignorance when we wish to collect specimens from volunteers who have been given virus but when we have no interest in similar materials from volunteers given no virus. Sometimes we collect specimens from the controls only to discard them in the laboratory. Sometimes we rely on the results of laboratory tests as a further extension of the "blind" procedure, for no one in the experiment knows whether volunteers who have been given a virus will or will not show evidence of being infected by it.

(5) A volunteer's symptoms and any physical signs referable to the upper respiratory tract are recorded daily on a standard form. The volunteer is observed for four days before inoculation so that we can obtain a "base-

line" of important clinical signs, such as the amount of
nasal secretion which is recorded in a semi-quantitative
way by the number of small standard paper handkerchiefs used each day. Those with known chronic or recurrent upper respiratory tract disease are excluded
before arrival at the Unit. Those with catarrh after a
recent cold or a high "baseline" of nasal secretion can
be excluded at the end of this quarantine period. Small
but significant changes occurring after inoculation can
then be detected. In the final assessment all the symptoms and signs are taken together. To use four or more
handkerchiefs above the baseline is a cardinal sign of a
mild cold; if additional symptoms are present or numerous handkerchiefs are used, then the condition may be
graded as a moderate or severe cold. If the symptoms
subside in 24 hours or are milder than this, the disease
is called "abortive" or "doubtful mild," and such cases
are scored as "no cold" in the final reckoning. (This is
done mainly because experience has shown that mild
symptoms occur from time to time in volunteers who
have been given noninfectious inoculum. This volunteer
technique was used first as an efficient means of studying laboratory fluids for the presence of a cold-producing
agent, and for this purpose it was necessary to be able
to produce a clear negative result with noninfectious
material even though occasionally the milder symptoms
of infection with a virus were passed off as not significant.) In addition, we usually disregard symptoms which
are not typical of colds. This cannot be done in all experiments, for sometimes an inoculum will give significant symptoms related to other body systems; for
example, diarrhea is produced by ECHO II virus, or
constitutional symptoms, like those found in severe

colds, may occur without the typical rhinitis. Such diseases have to be recognized as significant or not on other grounds, and the additional symptoms are recorded in the same way as the symptoms of typical colds.

All Kinds of Precaution

For thoroughness, the Common Cold Research Unit investigators went to great lengths to ensure success for their project. Intercurrent infections are inevitable if volunteers have contact with the general public. As a result, more volunteers had to be used to prove that a particular material is infectious. What concerned them was not the "taking of a cold" by those *inoculated* of the infectious material, but the "catching of cold" also by the *uninoculated* controls of a small percentage of the total group. Care had to be exercised to make sure they were working with infectious material. Why? Because in propagating viruses serially in man—and harvesting them as true infected secretion—additional unknown agents had to be screened out.

The following steps were taken to ensure some semblance of "reasonable isolation":

(1) Strict cleanliness. Rooms, bedding, household utensils, books and games were kept appropriately clean.

(2) Volunteers were kept thirty feet away from other persons in the open air.

(3) Volunteers were not allowed to enter any public place or a room occupied by another person.

(4) The clinical observations were made by staff members wearing masks and gowns.

It is clear, therefore, that isolation was indispensable.

Efforts to Study the Transmission of the Common Cold at the Common Cold Research Unit

The following is a list of the Common Cold Research Unit's assessment of how colds were transmitted:

(1) Colds seemed to be affected by all sorts of seasonal and individual response factors.

(2) Experimental evidence suggests that many of the airborne droplets produced in a sneeze start from the mouth.

(3) Volunteers caught colds in the same room as subjects with colds who were separated from them by a blanket hung across from wall to wall.

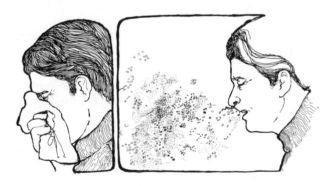

MAN SNEEZING—NOTE PARTICLES OF DIFFERING SIZES, MOST OF WHICH COME FROM THE MOUTH. HANDKERCHIEF STOPS ALL PARTICLES WHICH CONTAIN GERMS.

(4) Volunteers caught colds if they spent some time sitting next to others with colds.

(5) Volunteers spent months on a remote Scottish island and failed to develop colds when given experimental inoculum; they did develop colds when in contact with a man who had a naturally acquired cold and who was imported from the nearby mainland.

Children as Volunteers

In reviewing the work done with volunteers, I noted that none was done with children as volunteers. This seemed strange to me, since the research findings in England stated that *children caught more colds than adults*. However, in checking with Sir Christopher Andrewes, I learned that the reason children were not used as volunteers were:

(1) Children are liable to have more serious illness after respiratory virus infections; we don't want to do anyone any harm.

(2) Our volunteers come after having understanding of the nature of what they are volunteering for. Children could not understand this, and it would be ethically unjustifiable to ask anyone to volunteer for them.

(3) Our volunteers are at large and can take country walks but are "on parole" not to go near other people. This has worked well. We could not rely on children to obey such discipline strictly.

Dr. George Gee Jackson's Work at the University of Illinois

Dr. George Gee Jackson, and his associates, much like Dr. Tyrrell, worked with a large number of volunteers. Employing similar methods of clinical observation but different methods of isolation, both have shown that volunteers can be used for many purposes: the induction of colds by nasal secretions to demonstrate the presence of infectious agents not otherwise identifiable, and the demonstration that viruses, isolated from cases of respiratory disease, reproduced with disease after having grown in the laboratory.

Dr. Jackson pointed out that in some instances difference can be shown between the cause of illness and a virus isolated in tissue culture. In addition, alterations in the illness-producing capacity of some viruses have occurred on passage, in tissue culture.

In relation to the host factors, Dr. Jackson has pointed out that constitutional factors of the individual host, as tested in volunteers, contribute significantly to susceptibility and illness.

In the work of Dr. Jackson and his associates, it soon became apparent that secretions differed in infectivity and in the characteristics of the infection produced. None of the infectious secretions infected all of the subjects, and it was possible to identify certain host factors that influenced the development of symptoms. It was not possible, however, to induce increased susceptibility of the subjects by chilling them with controlled alterations of temperature and humidity. In further experiments, pooled human gamma globulin was shown to neutralize the infectivity of the nasal secretions, and volunteers were found to have specific immunity to reinfection three weeks or later after the initial challenge.

Regarding the nature of respiratory disease viruses as they occur in human nasal secretions, serologic and clinical data were presented to demonstrate two phenomena: (1) more than a single infectious agent may be present in nasal secretions during a natural cold, and (2) the disease-producing capacity of a respiratory virus may be appreciably altered by its passage in an alternative host.

Dr. Vernon Knight's Work in Bethesda, Maryland

Dr. Knight produces a standard infection in volunteers by use of an aerosol chamber. This aerosol method was useful for studying illnesses induced in volunteers by the Coe strain of Coxsackie A21. The incubation period ranged from two to three days, and men without preexisting neutralizing antibody had more severe infections, manifest by fever, myalgia and bronchitis, than those with antibody, in whom symptoms, if present, were limited to the upper respiratory tract. In other studies it was shown that volunteers without antibody to adenovirus types 26 and 27 responded to challenge with either of these agents by developing conjunctivitis and an antibody titer rise to both. The intestinal tract was found to be the site of a prolonged, asymptomatic viral infection in nonimmune volunteers. No evidence of clinical illness was induced in volunteers by reovirus types 1, 2, or 3. Volunteers infected with another reovirus type 1 strain, an isolate from cattle, also developed no illness; but they did show rises of antibody to reovirus types 2 and 3, as well as to the homotypic virus.

Opinions Regarding Volunteers

At the Conference on Newer Respiratory Disease Viruses held in Bethesda, Maryland on October 3, 4, 5, 1962, participants contributed additional observations and ideas in the discussion which followed, and the remarks themselves served to highlight the methodology discussed by the panel.[1]

I was impressed with their views on the use of volunteers, which views I shall present herewith.

Dr. D. A. J. Tyrrell and Dr. George Gee Jackson were asked to elaborate a bit on whether or not there is the need to isolate volunteers. (It is known that Dr. Jackson does not; Dr. Tyrrell does.)

Dr. Tyrrell pointed out that it all depends on what you want to do, and that in the course of their initial experiments at the Common Cold Research Unit they were trying to use as economical an experimental design as possible. In order to do what he was striving for he thinks a technique involving strict isolation of volunteers is needed and that was why Dr. Andrewes designed the setup that way.

Dr. Jackson pointed out that ideally one would like to be able to isolate volunteers, but it is not feasible in our society. He believes that isolation has the disadvantage that one cannot use large numbers of people. If you define antibody status, the susceptibility, the infectivity rate or the expected attack rate, you do not need large numbers of volunteers. He believes that if one can define as many variables as one knows about and set the experiment so that a small number of persons give the answer, then strict isolation of this small number is perhaps ideal. When one is dealing with a great many variables

---

[1]*The American Review of Respiratory Diseases* 88 (September 1963).

which can be neutralized insofar as one knows, only by statistical numbers, then Dr. Jackson thinks it impractical to try to isolate so many people, considering both expense and people's time. Therefore, there are some experiments that he thinks are preferable when performed on larger numbers of volunteers without the need for isolation.

Dr. Karl M. Johnson of the National Institute of Health, Balboa Heights, Canal Zone, took a different tack than that of Dr. H. G. Pereira of London, which was that under the conditions that prevailed in Salisbury, where he worked, it was very important in every single trial to have concurrent controls, as comparable as possible, with experimental volunteers. Dr. Johnson said he thinks the days for employing volunteers to gain some knowledge of whether or not a given new and unknown agent is a "respiratory pathogen" are numbered. He pointed out that to do a volunteer experiment costs a tremendous amount of money, and it costs even more when you decide in advance what sort of volunteer you want. He said it should be remembered that for most purposes it is generally not possible to get children for volunteers. Some of the reasons are legal; there are many social reasons why such studies in children have not been done to a great degree and are not likely to be done in the near future.

My Opinion Regarding Volunteers

In all the material I have read pertaining to experimental studies with volunteers, I have not found any mention of work done to determine the relationship between their diet and cold incidence.

It seems to me that this relationship is a most important factor in common cold research. If such studies were carried out, they would make the need for large numbers of volunteers unnecessary and thereby reduce the costs of experimental studies.

I recommend that future research groups bear this, as well as my theory of cold-causing foods, in mind and design their projects accordingly.

Holland's Research into the Common Cold

There is a generally accepted theory that a cold is "caught" by contact with one who has a cold. However, in a study, as reported in the *British Medical Journal,* January 25, 1958, 8,000 volunteers in widely scattered areas in Holland all had the same incidence of colds at the same time every year. Obviously, since they were in different parts of the country there was no contact between them.

My Interpretation

It is hard to imagine that each case in each area could somehow transmit his cold to other persons in a different part of Holland. Therefore, it follows that these colds were due to something other than contact. Though medical literature states that the "cold season" runs from October to April, and I agree that there is a high peak then, I have paid special attention to the fact that people catch colds 365 days a year. There is, therefore, a *daily* reason for the common cold. I have found that reason to be harmful foods with which I deal in this book.

7. My Research with Common Cold Victims

For thirty-five years through extensive reading and interpretive thought, I have found nutrition to be the determining factor in a person's state of health. In my search to find the cause of the common cold, I discovered, in addition to the common concept that an imbalanced diet is responsible for ill health, that faulty eating habits and the wrong preparation of food are at the root of many maladies (see Chapter 19).

During my lecture tours I constantly questioned people about their eating habits. I observed that there were some who seemed to sparkle with health. I learned from them that their diets included special health foods, some organically-grown produce, supplementary vitamins and minerals. Those whose health was poor and who were seeking help admitted to faulty diet.

There have been many books written as a result of laboratory tests, physical examinations, work with volunteers, etc. I do not minimize the merit of such works. However, my type of research has brought revolutionary results which are incorporated in my books.

It has been my experience not only with work on this book, but in preparing my other books, *Arthritis and Common Sense, Good Health and Common Sense* and *How I Stopped Growing Bald and Started Growing Hair,* to approach each problem involved through my own method of research. This entailed personal experimentation with all types of foods and liquids, and extensive questioning of people in an effort to find out first hand what I needed to learn to develop my theories.

My book, *How I Stopped Growing Bald and Started Growing Hair,* is proving helpful to many men and women. The top of my head was completely bald, but as a result of my regimen outlined in the book, I have grown a substantial amount of new hair in the past year. I have always had fringe hair around my ears but it is now quite thick. There are photographs on display in bookshops and health food stores showing me "before" and "after." There is a constant demand for *Arthritis and Common Sense* which is nearing a million sale. *Good Health and Common Sense* will very likely be brought forth soon in a revised edition.

I am not a doctor. However, I have had extensive experience with diet and nutrition. I constantly evaluate foods eaten by other people and myself to find out their relationship to the condition of the skin, sleeping habits, the functioning of the digestive system, as well as general well-being. My approach to problems of health is a creative one which has brought forth discoveries which can help mankind.

With regard to the common cold, during the early questioning of thousands of cold victims, after much study, I began to suspect that it was the *last course of the meal* that was the consistent troublemaker. It was the dessert, the sticky sweet. Fortified with this suspicion, I then proceeded to continue questioning people to confirm it.

There were those who had colds at the time of questioning, those who had recently recovered from colds, and those who had had only one or two colds during a period of as long as ten years or more.

In every case, I asked the person what foods he had consumed prior to a manifestation of his cold. However, one of the difficulties I encountered was that some of the people could not readily remember, as two to five days had passed since their colds had started. Therefore, I had to ask many questions until I found the information I sought.

I asked, "What day did you find that you had a cold and what time of the day was it?" Usually the cold victim reported that he found he had a cold in the morning of the day stipulated.

My next question was: "To the best of your recollection, what dessert did you eat at dinner the night before the day you realized you had a cold?" There were those who claimed they had had no dessert at dinner the night before.

I then asked what his main dinner course consisted of and where the meal was eaten. Was it in his home, a restaurant, a convention, a party, a group-gathering or at work? When this information was given, I again asked about the dessert.

In an effort to help each person remember, I mentioned various types of desserts which he may have eaten. If he still claimed he had had no dessert, I then asked what beverage he had had. Was there sugar or syrup in it? If it was milk, was it chocolate milk? If it was an after-dinner drink was it a sweet, sticky liqueur? If he had had no sweet beverage of any sort, I then asked whether he had spent the rest of the evening, after dinner, at home or at some outside activity and what he had eaten then. If he had not eaten a dessert any part of the previous night, I asked if he had had any sweet the morning and/or afternoon of the next day. If he claimed he had not, I asked him to try and recall if he had eaten a sweet at any point several days preceding his cold.

I found that a majority of the people I questioned *finally remembered* that they had eaten some kind of dessert at the evening meal or in the evening preceding the day they found they had a cold. A small number had done so the preceding day, and the smallest number several days prior. In most cases each one had eaten cake, cookies, pastry, sweet rolls or candy or drunk a sweet liqueur. Most desserts eaten were partly chocolate or of a sticky, sweet consistency. (I found that those who had had only one or two colds during the past ten-year period never ate or drank sweets of any kind.)

My next question was: "Did you eat the sweet in the presence of someone with a cold?" If he did not know, I asked whether there were a number of people present. In just about every case, I eventually found that there was someone present with a cold or who developed a cold the next day.

After compiling my findings it became evident to me that practically *all of the cold victims had eaten sweets twelve to seventy-two hours prior to the day they realized they had a cold and that they had done so in the presence of someone with an apparent or potential cold.*

After the cold victim had acknowledged eating a sticky sweet or drinking sweet liqueur in the presense of someone with a cold, I asked if he had felt a tickling in his throat thereafter and, if so, how much later. Invariably, it was felt *three to four hours after the consumption of the sticky sweet.*

I next asked when cold symptoms appeared. It was generally the next morning at which time he sneezed often, coughed and had either a stuffy nose or a watery nasal discharge. Also at the same time his throat was sore and his voice raspy.

I take exception to those who regard the nose as the initial area where the common cold starts. In my opinion the throat is the area where the infection starts. Through my research I learned that the common cold victims' throats *tickled first,* and then the next day there were symptoms of the cold in the nose and elsewhere. In Chapter 2, "The Major Cause of the Common Cold," I describe how the infection starts in the throat.

"How long did your cold last?" I then asked. The time varied from a day to two months or more. However, in most cases the cold lasted three to ten days.

I readily deduced that those whose colds had lasted only a day or two either had an allergy or their colds had been aborted. Those whose colds lasted a few days, the normal length of time, were asked if they had eaten sweets during that time. Some had had no sweets. Some admitted to having eaten sweets just once. Those whose colds lingered on beyond a week were, in all likelihood, reinfected with new colds because they had eaten sweets in the presence of someone infected with, what I assumed, was another virus strain and not the same one they had originally contracted.

However, there were those who did not eat sweets, yet their colds lingered on. I questioned them at length about their diet. I found they had and were still eating refined, devitalized and processed foods. Because of this the repair of the respiratory tract was slower, and the body could not develop antibodies to fight the replication of viruses.

I went back to cold victims I had interviewed the previous year and asked whether they had followed my suggested regimen of a diet containing more vital foods and had refrained from every kind of sweet. Those who had followed my regimen had not caught another cold. Those who had succumbed to the dangerous sweets suffered recurring colds.

I asked cold victims what they did to get relief from their colds. The majority reported that they took some form of cold remedy or aspirin. There were those who did not take any medication but drank large quantities of fruit juice. Some took large doses of vitamin C. Many stayed at home and kept warm for the first few days. Others drank hot toddies. Some used nose drops, cough syrups and gargled with salt water. Others used steam inhalation. A number felt the remedies they took made them feel somewhat better. They all agreed what they did were not cures and were aware of the fact that no cure for the common cold has been found yet.

Because there is such a scarcity of dietary literature a cold sufferer can follow in order to recover faster, the cold victims I questioned did not know how to help themselves through better nutrition. This is now available in Part V of this book.

As a result of the information gained from the foregoing interviews with common cold victims, the reader can readily recognize *how the common cold is caught*. I trust everyone will benefit from this knowledge, be free of colds and enjoy good health.

8. Does Cold or Chilling Produce Colds?

In the early part of my life, my parents bundled me up heavily when I went out during the cold, New England winters. They believed this necessary to avoid catching cold. I can remember wearing high-cut shoes laced all the way up to my knees. Even though they were waterproofed, my mother insisted I also wear rubbers. I wore a woolen scarf, woolen sweater, a heavy overcoat, woolen hat and earmuffs. Later, as I progressed to junior high and then high school, I shed at least 50 percent of the heavy clothing. Often I would be caught in stormy weather with very light clothing. But I recall that I did not catch cold as a result. I am sure that many readers who have lived in seasonal climate have gone through similar experiences.

I now live in Los Angeles, California, where the coldest temperature I have experienced is 38°. The evenings are much cooler than the days, but I dress the same day and night. Even so I have not caught colds. I have observed that, though the temperature here is warmer, people on both coasts get about the same number of colds each year.

It is the consensus among many people that colds come as a result of being chilled. However, there is no scientific proof to substantiate this belief.

I have always believed that feeling cold, in and of itself, does not result in catching cold. This has been borne out by tests made on human volunteers to find out whether being cold produces colds. There is extensive literature available on these experiments.

The experiments carried out by the Common Cold Research Unit in Salisbury, England, as recorded in *The Common Cold*, by Sir Christopher Andrewes, were as follows: In the first experiment, the Research Unit took three groups with six volunteers in each. They specially volunteered for the rather harsh treatment given them.

Three pairs received up their noses virus so diluted that the researchers expected it to produce very few colds.

Three pairs of volunteers took hot baths and thereafter stood about in bathing attire, undried, in a cool corridor for half an hour or as long as they could stand it. Then they were allowed to dress but still wore wet socks for some hours. Most of them had a considerable drop in body temperature and felt rather chilled and miserable.

The other three pairs received the dilute virus plus the special chilling treatment.

Chilling alone produced no colds. The group receiving virus alone developed two colds; those with chilling and dilute virus got four colds. This difference looked like something, but the numbers were too small to convince the Salisbury team. So they repeated the experiment in just the same way— and obtained the opposite result. The chilling alone was again not followed by any colds, but this time there were twice as many colds in the group with virus alone as in the group with chilling as well as virus.

In a third experiment on similar lines, the chilling consisted of sending the subjects out for a walk in the rain. They were not allowed to dry themselves for half an hour after their return, and, furthermore, the heating in their quarters had been turned off. Again there was no evidence that chilling had increased susceptibility.

Experiments on similar lines were carried out in Chicago by Drs. Dowling and Jackson and their colleagues. They used larger numbers of volunteers who were not held in isolation. . . . Groups of volunteers, who did or did not receive virus up their noses, were kept for four hours at a time at (1) a chilling temperature of 60° F. and an 80 percent relative humidity (RH) or (2) at a comfortable temperature of 80° F. with 30 percent RH or (3) at a really cold temperature of 10° F. and 80 percent RH. The last group only had to stand it for two hours. Those in the first two groups wore minimal clothing; those in group [three] wore street clothes. Most of the people in the first and third groups did quite a little shivering before they were liberated. They did not, however, develop more colds than those who were unchilled. The figures were 36, 32 and 39 percent for the three groups, the difference being regarded as without significance considering the numbers concerned.

. . . Because your socks are wet and you feel chilly, you think the wetness causes the cold which shortly develops. You do not consider the possibility that you felt chilly because the virus already had a grip on you. Plenty of people get their feet wet and get no cold and forget all about it. It has been recorded that soldiers in terribly cold and wet conditions in the trenches in the First World War showed no tendency to develop colds then, but were very apt to do so when back in comfort-

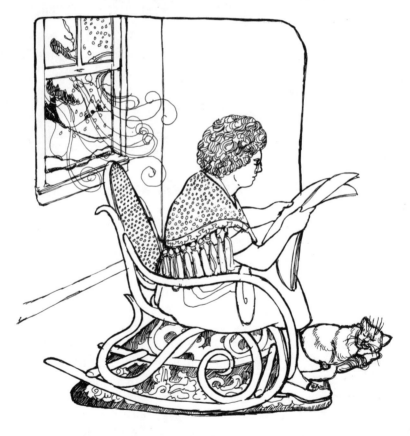

EXPERIMENTS HAVE PROVEN THAT CHILLING DOES NOT CAUSE THE COMMON COLD.

able billets. A point worth noting is that those who say that chilling starts off their cold usually state that symptoms develop within a few hours of the chilling. This is a very short time to allow virus infection to wake up and get going.

The second explanation, however, does allow that chilling might really start off a cold. It suggests that we did our tests on the wrong volunteers. Maybe chilling works, but only in people whose defenses are in a state of unstable equilibrium with a virus which they are harbouring, a virus which is just awaiting its chance. Chilling would then work but only sometimes, in some people. It seems necessary to postulate something of this sort if we are to have a reasonable explanation for the effect of weather, especially cold weather, on the incidence of colds. . . .

—From *The Common Cold*

The question of drafts in relationship to colds is worth considering. Again, I would like to point out that there are many people who seem to think there is more danger from localized draft on the body than from generalized chilling. However, there is no scientific proof to substantiate this.

Thirty years ago, medical literature contained a great deal of pro and con discussion on the danger and benefits of cold, fresh air. Efforts were made to approach this experimentally. It is regrettable that some of the people involved in this work were of the opinion that cold caused cold and proceeded to try and discover how it did so.

In the United States, about 1920, Drs. Mudd and Grant studied the effect of cooling parts or all of the body on temperature changes in the nose and elsewhere. Earlier belief was that chilling caused congestion and swelling of the nasal mucous membranes. However, they proved that chilling caused a reflex contraction of the blood vessels in the nose and throat which resulted in pallor due to lessening of their blood supply.

The experiments are outlined in *The Common Cold* as follows:

> . . . The experimental subjects were kept in a comfortably warm room and their normal clothes had been removed but they were "warmly wrapped in loose garments." They were chilled by removing the wraps with or without the application of cold wet towels to the back or playing the draft from an electric fan on the back. A simple apparatus applied to the inside of the nose enabled the doctors to measure changes in temperature. Chilling caused the nose temperature to fall rapidly, sometimes as much as 6° C.; after re-wrapping the subjects, it soon began to rise but was often not back quite to normal for half an hour or more. When the feet of the subjects were chilled by wrapping cold, wet towels and turning an electric fan onto them, the temperature in the nose fell, but only by 0.29° C. which was not very dramatic. It is recorded that one of the subjects in the above series of experiments developed a cold; he had not been kept in isolation, so the occurrences can hardly signify very much. Still, it is apparently the basis of the statement in a textbook on colds that "experiments have shown that when cold drafts of air are allowed to blow on the skin of healthy individuals the surface temperature of the mucous membrane of the mouth and throat is definitely lowered, and that following such change in temperature many of those subjected to the draft promptly develop symptoms of rhinitis.

Other experiments were carried on with forty-three volunteers to determine the effects of cold exposure on experimental rhinovirus infection. From the data on these cold-exposed volunteers and the controls, there was no difference between them which would suggest an effect of cold on the common cold.

I gathered this and other information on this subject from the *Medical News*, in an article entitled "Cold Doesn't Affect the 'Common Cold' in Study of Rhinovirus Infections." The three investigators who reported on their study initiated at the National Institute for Allergy and Infectious Diseases are R. G. Douglas, Jr., M.D., Baylor University; R. B. Couch, M.D., associate professor at Baylor; and K. M. Lindgren, M.D., National Institute of Health.

Dr. Douglas noted that, since earlier studies on chilling and the common cold, the importance of rhinoviruses as the major cause of common cold—at least in adults—has been established. In this study he described what was done: "Rhinoviruses were used to inoculate volunteers who were free of detectable antibody to this virus."

There were two methods used for cold exposure. In one, a volunteer was placed in "the Cold Room" which was cooled to 4° C. (39.2° F.), for one and a half to two and a half hours. In the other method, a water bath at the temperature of 33° C. (91.4° F.) was used for a similar period. The Cold Room was believed to be similar to short-term chilling experienced in natural circumstances. This experiment did not result in lowered rectal temperature, according to Dr. Douglas.

Further experiments were: Nine volunteers remained in the Cold Room for two hours, and eight controls stayed in a normal temperature. Three cold room volunteers and two

controls were given a calculated 0.1 infectious unit of rhinovirus by nose dropper or aerosol. This was the largest dose
given. All the individuals involved "caught cold." However,
with a dose ten-fold less, one of the three volunteers in the
Cold Room and none of the three in normal temperature
became infected. I found it very meaningful that, with the
smallest dose, none of the cold room or control volunteers
became infected.

Experiments were carried on with other volunteers, and
the results are reported in the article in the *Medical Times.*

Effect of cold during the course of illness was studied.
Three volunteers were immersed in the 33° C. (91.4° F.)
bath at the height of illness—about the third day—for periods
of two to four hours. As a result of this, there was no difference in their illness and that of other infected volunteers.

In the final study thirteen volunteers were exposed to cold
in the Cold Room and the Cold Bath during recovery from
infection with rhinovirus. Results were compared with those
of volunteers who had been inoculated with rhinovirus at the
same time but not exposed to cold. One cold-exposed volunteer, who had been in the bath, had a one-day relapse in
which there was nasal obstruction and discharge, malaise and
a cough. No relapses were seen among controls.

In a case of a volunteer who had been placed in the Cold
Bath at the height of rhinovirus illness, Dr. Douglas said:
"The course of his illness included lack of fever; the quan-
titative virus-shedding pattern and the antibody responses were
typical for rhinovirus infection (with or without cold exposure), except that this volunteer also failed to develop the
usual neutrophilic response. The other two volunteers who

were exposed to cold during illness also demonstrated typical infection and illness."

Dr. Douglas pointed out that, because cold will lower host resistance to some experimental infections in animals "it remains possible that more prolonged and more severe cold exposures may result in such an effect on humans." But, he added, conditions in these and previous cold and the common-cold studies have been arranged to be as close as possible to those found under natural circumstances.

Dr. Douglas concluded: "It seems unlikely that more severe or prolonged conditions would be encountered frequently."

Though, as already pointed out, one may think the combination of wetness and feeling chilly causes the cold which develops shortly thereafter, one should rather consider the possibility that he felt chilly because the virus *already* had a grip on him. I want to strongly emphasize that the feeling of chilliness comes *after* one is infected by the virus. *One of the first symptoms of a starting cold is chilliness.*

Once and for all, the reader can be free of the fear that cold and chilling can cause a cold, since, as pointed out, it has been proven scientifically that they do not.

9. Refrigeration, Air-Conditioning and Their Effect Upon People

In the previous chapter, there is scientific evidence that cold and chilling do not cause the common cold. However, since the researchers *did not* interview people at their work or homes as I have, I believe my findings will be of further value in establishing that cold and chilling do not cause the common cold. I interviewed the following groups in Southern California who work in cold-to-freezing temperatures or live and work where there is air conditioning.

Florists

The people who work in flower shops are not exposed to extreme changes in temperature, although they are subjected to possible chilling. Flowers are kept in a refrigerated room at a temperature ranging between 40° F. and 45° F. Many

of the women who work in florist shops said that as a pre-
caution they wear sweaters or knit dresses the year around.
The men, however, wear their regular clothes.

One florist said that should she catch cold she does not
lose her sense of smell and is able to enjoy the fragrance of
all the flowers.

Another florist said she and her husband never catch cold.
I asked whether they eat sweets and was pleased to learn they
do not.

I found with regard to colds among florists that there were
either none or an average of three or four a year.

Fruit and Produce Men

The men who work in fruit and produce are not exposed
to extreme changes in temperature, although they, too, are
subjected to possible chilling. There are two kinds of coolers:
one is for citrus fruit, apples and potatoes, where the temperature is set at 53° F.; the other is for celery, lettuce and
other greens, where the temperature is set at 48° F.

One manager I interviewed said that the men in his department spend on the average of an hour a day in the coolers. His record of colds had been one in three years. The
record of his men had been an average of two or three colds
a year. When I asked if he eats candy, he said "Very little,
only one candy bar a day." I asked whether he eats it at
work or at home, and he said, "At home." Here is a situation
where it is perfectly safe to eat candy without catching cold.
This man does not eat candy in the presence of anyone with
a cold. He lives alone.

He and the men in his department wear regular clothing

and put on a light coat or windbreaker when they go into
the coolers. However, he pointed out that there are many
times when they don't bother to put these on.

Butchers

The temperature in the room in which butchers cut and
trim meat is approximately 45° F. to 50° F. The temperature
in the freezer room ranges from 20° F. to 40° F. below zero.
The temperature in the storage room for meat is 35° F. to
40° F.

Since butchers are subjected to these *differing temperatures,*
I was interested in finding out whether there could possibly
be any relationship between this and their incidence of catching colds. Many butchers said that the varying temperatures
had no effect upon them and that they had not caught colds
any more often than people they know in other fields.

In questioning a meat manager, I learned that the fifteen
butchers under his supervision, who were subjected to the
extreme changes in temperature, had not caught any more
colds than employees in other departments of the supermarket.

Another manager said that at the time he first became a
butcher, he contracted a cold which lasted for four months.
However, subsequently, he had had just a few colds that lasted
only three or four days. I learned that his sweet intake had
been greater at the time he had had the prolonged cold.

A few members in his department had had colds which
had lasted two or three weeks. However, most of the other
butchers had had no more than three or four colds during
the year.

Butchers wear their regular clothes and, in some cases,

shirtless sleeves. At times when they go into the storage room, they may put on a light sweater. When they go into the freezer, they may put on a mackinaw with a hood.

Meat Packers

The temperature in a meat-packing cooler is between 28° F. and 38° F. The meat packers work all day in this room at this constant, cold temperature. They wear light sweaters or sweat shirts.

The manager of one packing plant said he had not caught a cold for years and that he was not at all affected by the change in temperature. The men in his department had had an average of two or three colds a year, which is lower than the percentage throughout the country. Consequently, it would appear that working a full day in a cold temperature did not cause colds. I asked about their diet and learned that they very seldom eat sweets; they prefer beer which they said relaxes them. This I found significant in evaluating the small incidence of colds among them.

Refrigerator Truckmen

The men who work on refrigerated trucks, known as "reefers," are subjected to extreme temperature changes. The temperature in the truck depends on what is being transported. For fruit, margarine and produce, the temperature is 50° F. For fresh meat, it is 28° F. to 32° F. For frozen meat and fish, it is 50° F. below zero. During the hot weather the great contrast of temperature outside and inside the truck does not affect the men.

The manager of a refrigerator-truck concern said that three of the ten people who work under his supervision had had colds that had lasted three to four months. However, the other seven had had colds that lasted only a few days to a week. I asked about their diet and learned that the truckmen who had been victims of colds that had lasted three to four months had eaten glazed doughnuts in the morning of each work day as well as candy early in the afternoon, which they felt gave them quick energy and kept them awake. I asked the manager for a record of his colds and learned he had had one or two in the previous year. He does not eat sweets. He and the men wear regular working clothes.

In reviewing the circumstances under which these men work, it would appear that though there are some who get prolonged colds, the reason for this is their diet and not the extreme temperature changes.

Air Conditioning

In interviewing people who live or work where there is air conditioning, I found that some get sniffles, and sneeze for a short time each day. However, they do not as a consequence develop colds. Those who had caught colds averaged about three or four a year.

Some claimed that their colds had lasted longer than average because they were exposed to air conditioning. However, I found, upon thorough questioning, that improper diet was at the root of this.

In further research with people who work and live where there is air conditioning, I learned that there were some who had caught summer colds. At first, I wondered whether the great contrast in hot temperature outdoors and chilling air conditioning might have some bearing on these summer colds. However, I realized, after some thought, that millions are subjected to this contrast, and there have not been consistent epidemics of colds during the summer.

I live and work where there is air conditioning. I find I sneeze occasionally several times a week when the temperature changes from regular to cold. However, the sneezing stops after a few moments. I do not develop colds. Incidentally, I very rarely catch cold, because I conscientiously avoid chocolate and sticky sweets when I am among people. Each day, I come in contact with many people, some of whom have colds.

Of particular significance is the fact that during an eleven-year lecture tour throughout the world, often traveling in air-conditioned airplanes, I did not catch cold nor miss giving a lecture. On the planes, the stewardesses offered many tempting chocolate desserts and chocolate after-dinner mints, which I refrained from eating. Were I not to observe what I have found to be the proper diet (see Chapter 20), I would definitely be vulnerable to the common cold.

Improper nutrition lowers the body's resistance so that when there is an infection the reparative process is slower. This occurs regardless of whether or not one works or lives where there is air conditioning.

Summation

My interpretation of the foregoing findings is that the people who are subjected to extreme temperatures or air conditioning do not catch more colds than the average person. I, therefore, conclude that those subjected to refrigerated temperatures or air conditioning had caught colds (as had the other thousands I had interviewed in all walks of life) because of the consumption of chocolate or sticky sweets in the presence of someone with a cold.

Those whose colds had lasted for weeks to months had been reinfected a number of times by new strains of viruses because they had continued to consume sticky sweets which had irritated the throat mucous membrane, thus making them vulnerable to each new virus attack. It is also important to know that when the body is stressed by a cold it has less ability to fight new cold viruses.

COLD TEMPERATURE DOES NOT CAUSE COLDS! IMPROPER DIET DOES! RESISTANCE TO THE COMMON COLD CAN BE BUILT WITH SOUND NUTRITION (SEE PART V).

---

10. Season and Climate

As people grow older, they dread the coming of winter because they feel it can bring poor health. They believe they are more prone then to joint ailments, poor circulation and respiratory illnesses such as the common cold. Winter is the most costly season of the year because of the frequent use of doctors, the purchase of heavier clothing, fuel to heat houses, and automobile accidents on icy and wet roads. Because of these disadvantages, many people move to warmer climates. For example, California has had a mass influx of not only senior citizens but people of all ages. They believe they will enjoy better health in the California sun. Others move to Florida, Texas or Arizona, also seeking health and longer life. However, those who try to escape from constant bouts with the common cold find that, though they now live

113

in a warmer climate, they still catch as many colds a year. The climate, therefore, is not the solution.

According to Sir Christopher Andrewes, in his book, *The Common Cold*:

> . . . As far as colds are concerned, there is a peak in the autumn, a relative absence of colds in early winter, another peak at the New Year and often a lesser one in March. Whether the viruses causing these different peaks are the same or different, we do not know. There may be cold viruses which, like influenza, prefer to operate about the New Year. There is a fair measure of agreement that it is a sudden change which tends to start up colds, rather than a particular level of temperature or other climatic factor. Sudden changes may be associated with a high incidence of colds even when they occur in the summer or under tropical conditions. . . .

I have also found in self-experimentation and interviews with people that season and climate are not the determining factors in causing the common cold. What can be partially causal is *sudden change* rather than temperature or climate. Further, from *The Common Cold:*

> A particularly careful study was carried out by Hope Simpson in his practice. He plotted cold-incidence against temperature. . . . The conclusion reached was that the results were most probably mediated through an effect on relative humidity indoors. Readings of humidity tell how much water-vapour there is in the air. The amount which can be held in the air varies greatly at different temperatures; the relative humidity (RH) or degree of saturation of the air with water-vapour is the thing which affects our comfort and [is] most worth our

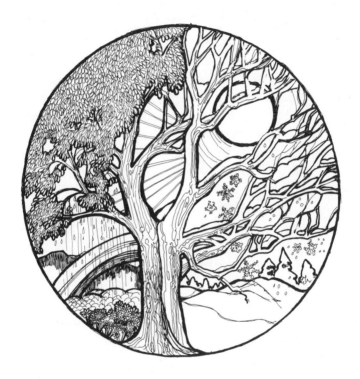

SEASON AND CLIMATE DO NOT START UP COLDS. SWEETS AND VIRUS
EXPOSURE DO.

attention. The RH out-of-doors tends to rise in the au-
tumn, but as soon as it grows cold and people light fires
or otherwise warm their houses, the RH indoors falls
rapidly. Hope Simpson found a correlation between incidence of colds on the one hand and the difference
between indoor and outdoor RH. As long as rooms were
artificially warmed, the opening of a door or window

did not manage to increase the RH. It does, however, rise when a room is full of people—and this presumably is when colds are apt to be caught, if caught they are. . . .

I repeat, season and climate do not trigger the common cold. I have already pointed out, in Chapter 2, my theory of what causes the common cold. It is important to be aware that when people gather together, particularly indoors, there can be a likelihood of catching the common cold if the mucous membrane of the throat has become irritated by eating chocolate or a sticky sweet in the presence of a common cold carrier.

It can prove very liberating to know that if you do not partake of chocolate or other sticky sweets in the presence of a common cold carrier you can live in any part of the world, during any season, any climate, any weather, indoors or outdoors, and you will not catch cold, providing you have been on a highly nutritional regimen which has built resistance against the common cold; this I promise!

Part III
Vulnerability

11. Smoking in Relationship to Catching Cold

As a result of studying smokers and nonsmokers and reading the important literature on the subject, I have taken the irrevocable stand, along with the surgeon general of the United States, that smoking is dangerous and can cause lung cancer. I am convinced that if one does not smoke it definitely helps prevent the common cold.

There is nothing so precious to a person as enjoying good health. One does not really appreciate it until he has a bout with any of the myriad illnesses that afflict mankind.

Sleeplessness is one of the great sufferings prevalent today. When the mind and soul cannot rest, one is unable to renew his energy to meet life. Sleeplessness can come from unconscious psychological causes. However, smoking is a conscious decision and act which the individual can control. One does not have to start smoking. One can stop smoking. It is common knowledge today that smoking leads to physical disaster.

In an article entitled "13 Million Quit Cigarettes," the author states that "more than 13 million Americans have successfully quit smoking cigarets since 1966, it was reported Wednesday at the first National Conference on Smoking and Health.[1]

> The statistic was described as a beneficial change in the national health picture so great that not even the most optimistic public health worker could have predicted it four years ago.
>
> Daniel Horn, director of the National Clearinghouse for Smoking and Health, said there are actually 4½ million fewer smokers in the United States now than were in 1966 despite an estimated population gain of more than 8 million.
>
> He said the tremendous changes in American smoking habits that these statistics represent are unique in the public health field.
>
> "I can't think of any comparison—in any way—in which so many millions of people have decided to stop doing something for their own medical benefit," he said.
>
> Horn said anticigaret TV ads sponsored by the various health agencies have helped, but that they merely gave impetus to something that began with the first cigaret-lung cancer scare of the 1950s and which continued with the surgeon general's report of 1964.
>
> In 1970, Horn said, 42 percent of American men and 31 percent of American women smoke cigarets, compared with 52 percent of men and 34 percent of women who smoked in 1966. . . .

---

[1]The *Los Angeles Times,* September 10, 1970 (copyright, 1970, *Los Angeles Times,* reprinted by permission).

A British epidemiologist said that despite optimistic statistics, the smoking of cigarets remains the biggest single problem in the entire field of preventive medicine in the Western nations of Europe and North America.

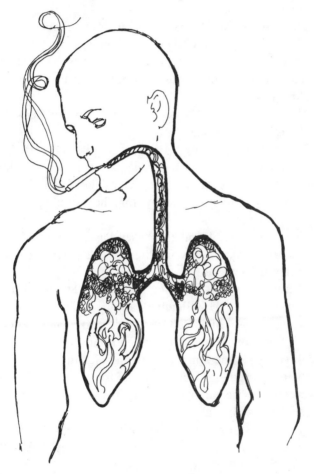

TOBACCO SMOKE PARALYZES THE NATURAL DEFENSES AGAINST THE COMMON COLD. SMOKERS HAVE A HIGHER PERCENTAGE OF COLDS. THIRTEEN MILLION AMERICANS HAVE QUIT SMOKING.

Dr. C. M. Fletcher, of the Royal College of Physicians, said the evidence against cigarets is so overwhelming that no doubt can remain in any "sensible person's mind" that they are extremely dangerous to life and health.

He said that a 35-year-old man loses about 15 minutes of life for every cigaret he smokes, and that the "worldwide epidemic of lung cancer" has been caused by cigarets much more demonstrably than by any industrial poison.

"Lung cancer is almost exclusively a smoker's disease," Dr. Fletcher said.

He said a huge proportion of British doctors have quit smoking in the last decade. As a result, the lung cancer death rate among physicians has fallen 35 percent, while remaining steady for the population as a whole.

The death rate from all causes has declined 12 percent among physicians compared to a 2 percent drop in the general population.

"Quitting cigarets is saving the lives of 80 British doctors every year," Dr. Fletcher said. . . .

"Cigarets as killers put cyclamates to shame," Foote said. (Emerson Foote, former chairman of the National Interagency Council on Smoking and Health)

"The government decided that if a man ate a few tons of cyclamates he might get cancer—and so off the market shelves came cyclamates.

"In contrast, on the conservative side about 25 million Americans now alive will die prematurely from the effects of cigaret smoking," Foote said.

He added that untold millions of Americans already in their graves were killed by cigarets.

Foote recommended that the federal government spend at least $100 million a year to educate the people about the dangers of cigarets.

He said that now is a time of "impending tragedy" for those who willfully persist in smoking, and described the money spent advertising cigarets as a "promotion of death."

Throughout this book, I have stressed that the common cold usually starts with a chocolate, sticky-sweet-irritated throat lining. However, I have not discussed that smoking, too, can irritate the throat lining. It has been proven that smoking causes hyperemia or congestion of the lining. That irritation is there day after day as long as the person smokes.

Medical literature points out that smokers have a higher percentage of colds than nonsmokers. Smokers are far more prone to catching cold, because the resistance of the entire body is lowered. The natural body defenses which fight virus infection are rendered useless when one smokes.

In an article in *Reader's Digest* of January, 1950, Roger William Riis states that smoking has a deleterious effect on lungs, on the heart, on stomach and digestion, on cancer incidence, on the blood pressure and blood vessels, on mortality rates and on the prowess of athletes. If you smoke a package of cigarets a day you take in 840 cubic centimeters of tobacco tar in a year. That means, he says, you have exposed your throat and lung tissue to 27 fluid ounces of tobacco tar containing benzopyrene. That is nearly a quart of liquid tobacco tar that your body must rid itself of.

The ugly, greasy tar that is left in your ashtray, on your fingers or in the filter of your cigaret holder is not nicotine. It is part of the "soot" that is left from the incomplete combustion of the tobacco—just as disagreeable and dangerous as the soot from your chimney. Many doctors agree that, as an irritant, it is more dangerous to heavy smokers than nicotine is.

Not only is there congestion of the throat lining, according to this report, but there is a high incidence of hacking coughs and tongue irritation. The consensus is that the way one smokes further effects the injury a smoker may suffer. The way you puff your cigaret, how long you hold the smoke when you inhale, how far down you smoke your cigaret— all have some bearing on how much irritation you are subjecting your throat tissue to. Rapid smoking, for instance, causes more irritation, because the smoke enters the mouth at a higher temperature.

Insurance companies make it their business to understand the problems and conditions of the nation's health. Their research (as published by National Underwriters Company in *Risk Appraisal*) indicates that smoking affects an individual's health. Insurance companies state that smokers have a 65 percent higher incidence of colds, 167 percent incidence of nose and throat irritation and some 300 percent higher incidence of cough.

It is a known fact that hundreds of thousands of people who daily take a coffee break light up a cigaret and simultaneously eat a candy bar. The common colds resulting from .eating the candy bars are also reflected in the statistics, though not acknowledged. It is of utmost importance to one's health to be aware of the *double danger of smoking and eating sweets*.

It cannot be said too often that smoking is injurious regardless of whether one is a light or heavy smoker. Smoking definitely increases complications in whatever illness a person is prone to. The membranes of the nose, throat, larynx and lungs are more directly exposed to smoke inhalation, and hence can become more irritated, than any other parts of the body. Therefore, nose and throat disorders, including the common cold, are more prevalent among smokers than nonsmokers.

There is no doubt that smoking destroys vitamin C and vitamin B which protect one from colds and other disorders. The candy manufacturer who claims he has enriched his product with vitamins C and B has not helped the consumer, as the candy is still the harmful substance which triggers the common cold.

A smoker's cold lasts longer than a nonsmoker's. The smoker is an easier prey for the sniffles, runny nose, fever, chills, coughs and hoarseness. The smoker's cold may well develop into serious complications, such as pneumonia, since the body's natural defenses against infection are paralyzed by the smoke.

A final word of warning. *Do not smoke, and do not eat chocolate or other sticky sweets.*

12. Do Doctors Catch Cold?

In the course of my research, I decided to investigate the seeming immunity of doctors to the common cold. Obviously, if I could discover how doctors avoid catching cold, it would be another clue in solving the mystery.

When I think back on my married life, I recall that the family doctor came to our house everytime our children ran a high fever accompanying their colds or my wife had severe episodes of the common cold or "strep" throat. I always marveled at how it was possible for our doctor to avoid catching my family's colds.

What is this seeming immunity that doctors have? Do they take cold and flu shots prior to the "cold season"? I know many people who had taken shots but, nevertheless, caught colds or the flu. Therefore, shots are not the answer. As for a "cold season," I have observed that people catch colds in

the summer as well as the winter. The doctor, therefore, is
exposed to cold victims all year around.

In the course of a day, the doctor sees many patients with
cold viruses. Approximately 10 to 20 percent of his patients
are victims of the common cold. He may see some patients
only when they are in an advanced stage of the common cold.
The doctor may even be a carrier of the common cold virus
himself. Why has he not caught a cold? Obviously, with such
exposure, the doctor is more vulnerable to the common cold
than any other person. In addition, doctors are subjected to
sudden changes in temperature when making house calls as
they get in and out of heated or air-conditioned cars. As a
rule, when they have heavy patient loads, they do not take
time out to eat a meal. All of this would seem to make the
doctor especially vulnerable to the common cold. Yet, in
many cases, they do not succumb.

Throughout the centuries doctors have worked amongst all
kinds of epidemics, of which some were infectious and some
contagious. It goes without saying that the doctors took whatever precautionary steps they could to avoid contracting the
diseases they were working with. In some cases certain diseases have now been brought under control by sterilization
and immunization. However, there still remain virus diseases
which develop into epidemics. One of these is the common
cold, which recurs year after year. It attacks entire schools,
entire military installations and entire communities. Still, most
doctors remain free of it.

What can we learn from a doctor's way of life that gives
him this seeming immunity to the common cold much of the
time? Most doctors know scientifically that chocolate is harmful to one's health, and they tell their patients to refrain from

it to avoid the many illnesses it can cause. A high percentage of doctors, of course, do not eat chocolate and chocolate-laden sweets, not only for health reasons, but because they do not want to gain weight. They know their appearance must set a good example for their patients.

I BELIEVE THE REASON MOST DOCTORS DO NOT CATCH COLD IS THAT THEY DO NOT EAT CHOCOLATE OR OTHER STICKY SWEETS! THOUGH THEY ARE CONSTANTLY IN THE PRESENCE OF PEOPLE WITH COLDS, THEY DO NOT BECOME INFECTED, AS THEIR THROATS ARE NOT IRRITATED FROM SWEETS.

On the other hand, there are some doctors, as well as nurses, who catch the common cold. Those who are afflicted have, somewhere in their busy schedule, picked up a chocolate bar possibly as a means of getting some quick energy. It is also quite likely that the doctors who catch colds eat chocolate or other sticky sweets at home when a member of their family is a victim of the common cold. Nurses have a great potential for the common cold because they are generally given boxes of chocolates as gifts, and they also eat their patients' candies.

To sum up: There is no magic to the doctor's seeming immunity to the common cold. It is a matter of his keeping his throat lining free of chocolate or other sticky sweets when he is in the presence of victims of the common cold. In this way, he avoids catching the common cold. This, then, creates the doctor's seeming immunity.

I hope the layman will realize now that he, too, can acquire this enviable "seeming immunity" and be free of colds.

13. Infants' and Children's Vulnerability to the Common Cold

From *Parents' Magazine,* January, 1966, in an article entitled "When Your Baby Catches Cold," by Dr. Carl A. Holmes, pediatrician, I have gathered comprehensive information regarding the problems of the common cold that face the infant.[1] Dr. Holmes points out that during the first few weeks of life infants seem to have a natural immunity to respiratory infection. On the other hand, as infants grow older, they do catch cold.

At the outset, I should like to establish why I believe this condition exists. The basic reason why babies catch cold as they grow older is that their diet changes radically. The infant that is breast-fed does not catch cold, because, in my

[1]This article is reprinted in Dr. Holmes' book, *Letters to Tricia* (Los Angeles: Sherbourne Press), and is used by permission of the publisher.

opinion, the mother's natural milk is pure. In addition, it is an established medical fact that mothers pass antibodies to their babies through breast-fed milk. It has also been found that antibodies can be transferred from the mother's blood-stream through the placenta to the fetus. The newborn infant, therefore, is immune to respiratory diseases the first few weeks of life.

On the other hand, an infant whose formula contains sweet, sticky corn syrup is much more vulnerable to catching the common cold if a cold virus is present. When the breast-fed baby is weaned, his new diet very often includes sweets. It is then that he becomes susceptible to the common cold.

As the baby begins to walk and talk, he is usually given a new variety of sweets such as cookies, frosted cakes and candy. At this juncture the child's vulnerability to the common cold is greatly increased. As I have already mentioned, one of the all-time favorite, but dangerous, sweets given to the child is the lollypop, which causes irritation of the throat, the trap for the common cold virus. As long as there is a lollypop, and it is consumed, you can be sure the child will be vulnerable to the common cold.

Going back to the article, Dr. Holmes points out that a baby, like a growing child or an adult, is more susceptible to a cold during the winter months, for that is the time when airborne viruses which cause colds and similar infections are most prevalent. But just being exposed to a virus is not enough to start a cold. Another element is needed—a lowering of general bodily resistance to infection. If a child gets overtired, his resistance may be lowered. If he gets chilled or overheated, he may more likely succumb to a cold virus.

I should like to repeat here my warning about the dangerous lollypop and other sticky sweets.

Once a baby catches cold his problems multiply rapidly. Dr. Holmes points out:

> As his nasal mucous membranes swell and mucus accumulates in his nose, he will breathe noisily and his nose will begin to run. Since a baby won't breathe through his mouth until his nose is completely blocked, he will snort and snuffle until the blockage becomes so extreme that no air at all gets through.
>
> He'll sneeze and act sick and weak. He may run a fever which can get quite high. Usually fever stays under 102° F. with a simple cold, but it may run up to 104°.
>
> As the baby's cold progresses, he'll begin to cough. Dry at first, the cough will become loose and rattling later on. Incidentally, after the baby coughs up mucus from his chest, he normally swallows it. A large part of the contents of a baby's stomach is made up of swallowed mucus from the nose and lungs whether a baby is sick or not.
>
> The runny and obstructed nose, the cough, and the other symptoms usually continue for four or five days before they begin to decrease. Then the fever disappears, the nose stops running, and the cough comes more rarely. The baby will begin to show more interest in food again and act more like his normal self. All symptoms of an uncomplicated cold will have disappeared about ten days or two weeks after its onset.
>
> When a baby does catch cold, his misery shows. He will fuss more than usual and his appetite will decrease.

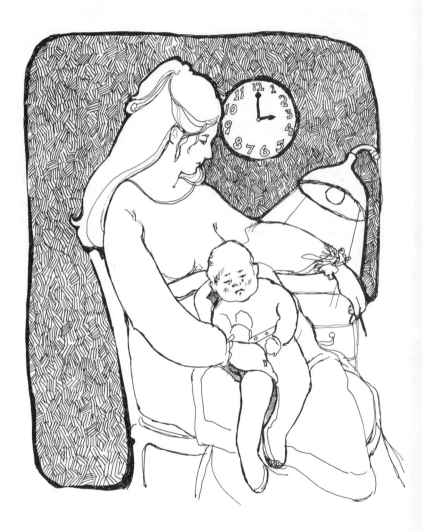

AN INFANT SUFFERING FROM THE COMMON COLD AS A RESULT OF
SWEET, STICKY SYRUP IN HIS FORMULA.

Since he'll probably eat less he may not have as much waste to pass. However, this does not mean that he will be constipated; the stools may be of normal consistency. . . .

With regard to protecting a baby from catching cold, Dr. Holmes states:

You can try to avoid exposing him to anyone who has one, but this can't always be done, for the infectious period begins slightly before the symptoms are noticeable. When another member of the household comes down with a cold, it is already too late to avoid exposure.

I would like to add my viewpoint. If a member of the family has a cold, which is apparent or not, the baby will probably not contract it if he is kept away from *every* form of sweets and if there is no physical contact with the common cold carrier.

It goes without saying that the reverse is true. If the baby has a cold, because he has been given sweets possibly by a thoughtless baby sitter or a doting grandmother, the parents should refrain from eating sweets so as to avoid catching the baby's cold. If the parents do not heed this and catch cold, the baby is then subjected to potential reinfectivity of another virus strain from the parents. Such a cycle of colds can continue for an extended period of time if sticky sweets are eaten.

Other measures to protect the baby, as recommended by Dr. Holmes, are:

Provide him with a good diet, supplemented by vitamins, seeing to it that his schedule provides both exercise and rest, keeping the temperature of your home to a comfortable 68° to 72°, and dressing him neither too warmly nor too lightly. A baby needs no more clothing outdoors in the winter than you do. In short, try to avoid lowering his resistance. . . .

In general, treatment consists of relieving cold symptoms by adding moisture to the air with a vaporizer and by taking aspirin, antihistamines and other medicines. . . .

Your doctor may or may not prescribe nose drops. If he does, he will recommend only those that contain no oil. Oily nose drops are particularly dangerous to babies and young children because if they should be inhaled into the lungs they may cause pneumonia.

One of the most important aids in the treatment of almost any respiratory disease, including the common cold, is a vaporizer. The nose is supposed to moisten and filter the air we breathe. When these functions are interfered with by disease, the unconditioned air taken into the chest irritates whatever passage it strikes. One result is a cough.

A vaporizer conditions the air by warming and moistening it and by filtering out dust. If it's kept running all night a vaporizer will put a gallon or more of water into the air. It will be just as effective in a corner of the room as it would be near the crib, so keep it safely out of the way.

During the early stages of a cold, when a baby loses his appetite, give him what he will take readily, but don't try to force him to eat. Fluids of almost any kind are good for him. However, don't let him fill up on milk, since a young baby, who has been eating solid foods for a short time, may get back into the habit of drinking milk as his sole food. It is better for him to get a little hungry as he gets past the worst stages of the cold so that he'll eat solids again.

Rest is advised for anyone with an infection. The sick baby will rest better if he is near his mother; so don't feel that a baby with a cold has to stay in his crib. He may be quieter in his carriage in the living room near his mother than off in his room in bed.

Dr. Holmes asks some leading questions:

Why do children catch so many colds? Doesn't a cold produce any immunity? Of course the common cold does produce antibodies which will protect the child from colds caused by the same virus. But the protection lasts only for a month to six weeks and the antibodies aren't effective against other strains of cold virus. . . .

Here, I should like to interject that children catch colds very often, because they eat sweets very often. In my opinion, antibodies produced by a common cold will last longer if the throat is kept clear of sticky sweets and the diet contains thoroughly healthful foods.

Dr. Holmes goes on to say:

There are two periods when it seems that children have one cold after another. Both are at times when they are suddenly exposed to many new people—about two-and-a-half to three, when they begin to play with other children, and again when they first go to school. Gradually, as children grow older, they become increasingly resistant to colds. . . .

I should like to add, for example, that, while celebrating their birthday parties, many very young children, whose

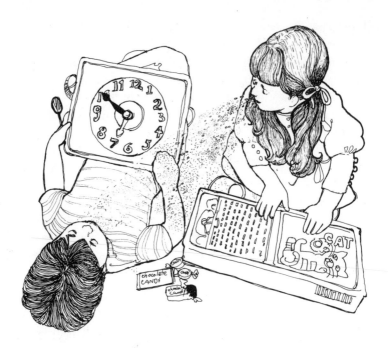

POTENTIAL MEANS OF TRANSMITTING VIRUS INFECTION IF SWEETS
ARE EATEN.

throats are irritated from sweets and who are in the presence
of one or more cold-carriers, will usually catch cold. The age
of the child is not the factor; playing with other children is
not the factor; starting school is not the factor. What is the
common cold-causing factor is the child's eating sticky sweets
in the presence of a viable, virus cold carrier.

Back to Dr. Holmes:

> . . . Though colds are unpleasant they're not serious as
> long as they remain uncomplicated. However, more seri-
> ous infections—ear and sinus infections, and pneu-
> monia—all usually begin with a cold; so consult a doctor

when a young baby gets a cold, and tell him promptly about any variations in a cold's usual course. Variations may include: an unusually high fever; any fever at all after the first five days; a cold which hangs on for over two weeks with a delayed appearance of discharges from the nose; earache; sore throat; pain in the face or chest. . . .

I have quoted Dr. Holmes so fully because I feel he has made a pediatric contribution of importance. I agree with him that "the more you know, the less upset you will be when the classic symptoms appear. Even with an ordinary cold, which will get better anyway, it helps to know what to expect."

Although this book explains how the common cold is triggered, unfortunately there will be those who will not take heed. Beyond the pleasure from eating something sweet, beyond the temptation and craving for sweets, there is the additional problem—children want what other children have. This has always been so. As a consequence, the inevitable reality is that children will eat sweets and will catch colds unless the parents are aware of the danger and *prevent them from eating sticky sweets.*

14. Adults' Vulnerability to the Common Cold

In my research concerning adults' vulnerability to the common cold, I found that parents of small children have more colds than adults without families. One reason is they are exposed to their children who are more prone to the common cold than adults (see Chapter 3). (However, I raise the point again here since it relates to the vulnerability of the parents in the family.) Another reason is that when parents make themselves vulnerable to the common cold virus by consuming throat-irritating sweets while their children are common cold victims, they—the parents—will in all likelihood catch cold.

Adults without children can also become vulnerable to the common cold if their resistance is low due to improper nutrition. (See Chapter 19.) Also, of course, they will be prone to the common cold if their throats are irritated by sweets while in the presence of a common cold victim.

Were an adult to take time out for a physical self-examination, he might discover symptoms in himself which are a result of an improper diet which at the same time makes him vulnerable to the common cold. Some manifestations are poor facial color, dull hair, persistent dandruff, dry skin, nails which break easily, absence of wax in the ears, pouches under the eyes, brown spots on the hands, white speckling on the palms of the hands, enlarged pores on the face, serrated edges of the tongue, fissuring of the center of the tongue, discoloration of the tongue, scaliness of skin on knees, ankles and elbows, and constipation. (See Chapters 18 and 20.)

A person's prescribed way of life often affects his vulnerability to the common cold:

A diabetic, by giving up sweets completely, becomes far less vulnerable to the common cold. However, if he eats sticky, artificially sweetened substitutes which irritate his throat, he will be vulnerable to the common cold.

The alcoholic is very prone to catching the common cold, as he usually does not eat a well-balanced diet. As a matter of fact, the confirmed alcoholic goes for days, at times, without eating at all. He has absolutely no resistance to any virus infection. When he catches cold it lingers for weeks at a time, because he has no recuperative powers. Frequently, when the alcoholic struggles to give up drinking, he craves sweets. Though his health will improve from abstinence of alcohol, with the consumption of sweets in the presence of a common cold victim, he will nevertheless become vulnerable to the common cold.

A person who has a tendency to put on weight will give up high calory desserts, and since there is an absence of sweets in his diet, he will be far less vulnerable to the common cold.

An adult who is on a low cholesterol diet has had to give up dairy products, fatty meats, nuts and sweets. Because of the absence of sweets in his diet, his vulnerability to the common cold is lessened.

In an article entitled "The Common Cold and Common Cold-Like Illnesses," Dr. John H. Dingle states that "the number of annual colds does decrease with increasing age.[1] I go along with this concept, as I have observed that people eat more wisely and consume fewer sweets as they grow older. This is the important, determining vulnerability factor regardless of one's status or age.

---

[1]*Medical Times* 94 (February 1966).

Part IV
Remedies

15. Recommended Self-Care of the Common Cold

In an article entitled "Education for Self-Care of the Common Cold," Dr. Douglass S. Thompson points out that medically approved, standard self-care methods of treating the common cold among college students at the University of Pittsburgh *reduce physicians' work loads by about 20 percent, thus enabling them to devote more time to doing a better job on other problems presented by students.*[1] Dr. Thompson is medical director, Student Health Service, University of Pittsburgh, Pittsburgh, Pennsylvania.

Dr. Thompson states:

People confronted by symptoms of illness or by injuries must make judgments as to whether they should

---

[1]Published in the *Journal of the American College Health Association* 14, no. 3 (February 1966), and quoted by permission.

or should not seek professional attention. Drs. White, William and Greenberg reported in 1961 that approximately one-third of such persons over a one-month time span seek professional attention. . . .

I believe that people should (and must) make self-judgments throughout their adult lives about when they should or should not seek professional attention for a medical episode, especially for those episodes that are recurrent in their lives and that are by nature short-lived, for which only symptomatic treatment is available, and are not helped any more by professional attention than by self-care. The common cold is the outstanding example of an illness that fulfills these criteria. . . .

The article says that a student first becomes aware of the existence of a recommended program when he or she registers at the Student Health Service to see a physician.

At the registration counter there is a sign inviting him, if he is there because he has a common cold, to consider the possibility that he may be able to care for this illness himself and therefore may not need to see the doctor. If he elects to investigate this suggested approach, he would then read a brochure entitled, "Colds—Sore Throats—What to do About Them." (There are numerous copies in the waiting room.) He reads [one] while waiting to see the doctor. This means that he will not lose his place in line (and usually this three-page brochure can be read more than once while waiting to see the physician, especially during the "cold" season). The brochure endeavors to get across the following points:

(1) Most (97 percent) respiratory tract infections

among otherwise healthy college students are upper respiratory tract infections.

(2) Most (90 percent) upper respiratory tract infections are caused by one or more of some 70 different viruses. These infections are referred to as colds or common colds.

(3) The symptoms of a cold at its various stages are one or more of the following: running or stopped-up nose, headache, sneezing, watering of the eyes, mild to moderate sore throat, hoarseness, mild to moderate nonproductive cough, fatigue, and generalized sick feeling (malaise) with or without a mild to moderate sensation of fever. These symptoms last from 3 to 14 days.

(4) The symptom period cannot be shortened, because there are no specific anti-cold-virus medications. Antibiotics (including penicillin) and sulfa preparations are of no benefit.

(5) Treatment is therefore limited to efforts to suppress the symptoms and make the victim more comfortable while the disease runs its course.

The need, the brochure goes on to say, is to diagnose the illness correctly. The patient is then asked a series of self-answerable questions similar to those the physician would ask in his differential diagnosis approach.

There are special questions relating to sore throats. All of these questions are designed to distinguish colds from bacterial and lower respiratory problems and to identify persons who have had streptococcal, respiratory allergy, or ear problems in the past or who have a significant chronic disease. The patient is also given an opportunity to take his own temperature. If the answer to the various questions is no and if the temperature is not over 99.4°F. (an arbitrary figure with a hoped-for high degree of sensitivity that will identify false positives but not false negatives), the student is informed that the illness is almost certainly a common cold and that the treatment is symptomatic only.

He may then elect to take the appropriate symptomatic treatment along with an instruction sheet. If so, he records on a master list his name, student status, temperature reading, and medication taken. He may elect to see the physician anyway. In either event, he is encouraged to return if his illness does not seem to progress favorably.

The symptomatic medications offered are 0.25 percent neosynephrine nose drops, Sucrets, salt for gargles and aspirin. The instruction sheet [see "Treatment of Common Cold"] details the use of these and offers general comments about fluids, rest, good hygiene, and, of course, smoking! It also points out that thermometers and all of these medications are readily available in drug and other stores without a prescription. It emphasizes that symptomatic medications are largely a matter of personal preference based on personal experience and suggests certain principles to keep in mind when selecting medications for a cold. . . .

Because I feel that Dr. Thompson's recommendations for the treatment of a cold will prove helpful to the reader, they are quoted herewith in full:

TREATMENT OF COLD

(1) For your feeling of tiredness, headache, malaise, chilliness, and feverishness:
Two aspirin tablets (a total of ten grains) every three

to four hours—you may chew these for slightly faster action.

(2) For your uncomfortable throat and cough:

(a) Hot (about as hot as you can tolerate) salt water gargle at least four times a day (ordinary drinking glass) with either a half teaspoon of salt or two 1.0 gram salt tablets dissolved in it. Gargle with head well back and do not swallow the gargle solution.

(b) Sucrets—analgesic throat lozenges. Suck them slowly and use as needed to reduce throat irritation. Actually, any hard candy [see note below] will provide more-or-less similar relief.

(3) For your running and/or stuffy nose:

Neosynephrine nose drops (0.25 percent concentration)—use approximately five drops in each nostril four times a day. Tip head well back, insert the drops, breathe in through your nose while holding head back long enough to give them a chance to get back to your throat. If you are gargling, gargle before using nose drops.

(4) For all of your symptoms:

(a) Drink a glass (eight ounces) of some liquid every hour.

(b) Avoid air with a low humidity content if you can.

(c) Get an extra amount of sleep and rest and avoid frivolous activities.

(d) Practice good hygiene with respect to others.

(e) Be patient and maintain good humor.

(f) Stop smoking while you have a cold (perhaps stop forever!).

. . . Medications for which you may have a personal preference are available at all drug stores without pre-

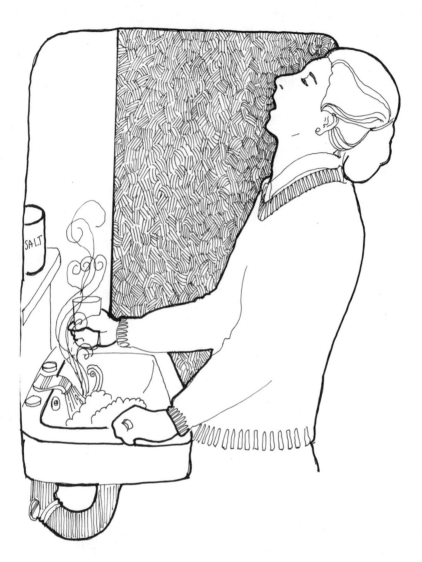

GARGLE WITH HOT SALT WATER (½ TEASPOON SALT), AS HOT AS YOU
CAN TOLERATE, AT LEAST FOUR TIMES A DAY FOR UNCOMFORTABLE
THROAT AND COUGH.

scription (as is a thermometer, which you should have for your personal future use). Any medication you use for the symptomatic treatment of your cold should be, in the last analysis, a reflection of your personal choice, since their only purpose is to make you more comfortable. Many are available, as you know. Several principles to be kept in mind when selecting medication for your cold are: do not use antibiotics in any form; nasal drops and sprays should be water based; your cough, although annoying, if productive of sputum may be helping you by reducing or eliminating secretion collecting in your trachea and lower respiratory tract—so such a cough should not be suppressed too much, if at all. . . .

Note—Hard candy should not be used for throat irritation because it most likely consists of sweet, sticky substance which will increase the possibility of reinfectivity.

The regimen outlined by Dr. Thompson for self-care treatment is practical knowledge gleaned from years of medical experience. Certainly aspirin and hot, salt water gargling will do much to reduce the uncomfortable symptoms of a common cold. As for liquid intake every hour, this is certainly sound advice, because the body can become dehydrated during the common cold. Another point is that during hot weather a cold sufferer requires more liquid than usual because of greater dehydration.

With regard to liquids, I want to emphasize strongly that the cold sufferer should not partake of any *soft drinks* at all (this includes all diet-type colas even if they are sugar free). Also, he should avoid frozen or canned fruit juices. The reason for my strong objection to these liquids is that they are devoid of enzymes which are needed to repair the body. Soft drinks do not have natural minerals nor natural carbohydrates. These elements are needed in the reparative process of tissue that lines the nose and throat and which becomes inflamed during a seige of the common cold. I recommend hot liquids such as herb teas be drunk during a cold, also fresh fruit juices at room temperature. As I have already pointed out (but it can bear repeating) it is preferable to drink hot liquids rather than cold, since the heat is soothing and prevents internal thermal shock, and I emphasize, drink liquids only on an empty stomach.

Here are some excellent recommendations for self-care when one has a cold:[1]

(1) Maintain an adequate, nutritious diet, including, of course, your vitamin supplements. Eat lightly if you will, but eat.

(2) Stay home and rest. This doesn't mean you have to "take to the sick bed." But take it easy. Lie down when you feel like it. Stay warm. Don't expose yourself to sudden changes of temperature.

(3) If possible, keep your distance from other members of the family so you won't spread the infection. Keep your own towels separate and away from others. Don't leave your dishes where a child might eat or drink out of them. Keep a paper bag near you for used tissue after you blow your nose.

(4) Blow your nose gently, with both nostrils open. A puddle of warm water held in the palm of the hand and sniffed in gently will flush out excess mucus without irritating tender nasal membranes.

---

[1]*Prevention,* February 1970, (quoted by permission of Rodale Press, Inc.).

(5) A moist atmosphere is particularly important when you are fighting a cold. You want to give the defense mechanisms of your respiratory system every help. A small vaporizer that can be purchased at the drugstore does a good "spot" job by the bedside or favorite chair.

(6) Avoid over-the-counter remedies. They won't cure you and they may very well do harm.

My recommended regimen to aid recovery and build resistance against the common cold is covered in Chapters 18 and 20. If these recommendations are followed, it will mean faster recovery, strengthened defenses and a healthier body, which can resist the common cold.

16. Comparative Treatment of the Common Cold

Since every doctor has his own method of dealing with his patients, I thought it might prove of interest and value to interview three different men in the medical field, posing pretty much the same questions regarding the common cold, and see wherein they agree or differ.

Interview with an Allergist

In questioning a West Coast doctor, who is an outstanding allergist, regarding the common cold and his treatment of it, the following are the results:

As to what percentage of his patients that catch cold come specifically to be treated for the common cold, he said that 90 percent who catch cold come in. He finds that 10 percent of those who come in thinking they have a cold, instead have some variety of allergy. He pointed out that there are many other people who do not go to a doctor when they have a cold unless there is a complication.

With regard to the percentage of colds that are upper respiratory and lower respiratory, he answered that there are more upper respiratory colds; he estimates they are five to one.

I asked what treatment he prescribes for a cold, and he pointed out that in acute cases he gives massive doses of vitamin C. Vitamin C works as a suppressive at first and then knocks out the cold. He claims that a virus cold can be aborted with large doses of vitamin C. It is his assumption that vitamin C kills the virus. However, he has done no laboratory testing as he could not get the facilities. In his extensive experience and success with patients, he is convinced that vitamin C is the answer.

In discussing how many colds are due to virus as compared to the number due to allergy, he said that probably 50 percent of colds are allergy in origin. He has found that there are people who think they have colds but instead have an allergy to cold temperature and cold drafts; they have not contracted a virus; they seem to be hypersensitive to change in temperature. Further he said that when a person has an allergy it produces a lesion. It is released from some of the mast cells. Histamine dilates the blood vessels. Histamine can cause the tissues to swell. Water-logging results and produces irritation which leads to sneezing. This then is interpreted as a common cold. You can differentiate, he continued. If the patient doesn't have a fever or sore throat it is less likely to be a virus. Further differentiation can be determined by a smear to pick up the presence of eosinophils which are an indication of allergy.

When asked what can precipitate an allergy, he said foods

such as wheat, eggs, milk, chocolate, corn, yeast and pork can, when there is an inherited enzyme deficiency or block.

What is the main symptom he looks for in determining therapy, I asked. If it is a lower respiratory infection, he said, he prescribes an antibiotic. If it is an upper respiratory infection, he doesn't prescribe an antibiotic unless the mucus is yellow or green. In all cases he prescribes massive doses of vitamin C.

I asked when he prescribes bed rest, and he said *only* if the patient feels sick enough. Mostly, he does not like bed rest for his patients.

With regard to supplements, he said he "covers the water front." They are prescribed as a preventive. He prescribes vitamin C to be taken indefinitely, as it raises resistance to respiratory diseases. A significant point he made parenthetically is that a postnasal drip, in many cases, is due to a food allergy.

When I asked if he prescribes eliminating specific foods from the diet, he said he finds it helpful for the patient to go on a diet of juices for 24 to 48 hours. Specifically they are carrot juice, unsweetened apple juice, unsweetened grape juice and freshly squeezed orange juice.

When I raised the subject of smoking in relationship to a cold, he said very definitely if one doesn't smoke it will help prevent a cold. The reason smoking causes colds is that it partially paralyzes the cilia—an important defense against virus infection. Smoking interferes with the defensive mechanism of the polys. Further, the gaseous components of the cigaret smoke, primarily the cyanide and acrolein, cause trouble as they destroy the efficiency of the white blood cells.

I asked what he thinks the basic cause of the common cold is, and he listed poor diet as the primary one; then chemicals in food, water and air; stress of other types; and breakdown of immunity. When I pursued poor diet as the cause, he said unquestionably a large percentage of colds is due to poor diet.

As to why children catch more colds than adults, he explained that specific immunity mechanism is not built up, as the children have not encountered as many viruses as frequently as adults have.

Why are more colds caught in mid-winter than at any other time, I asked. He said there are about the same number of colds in the spring, fall and winter. The reasons: people spend more time indoors and in larger groups. Then, too, viruses are more active during these seasons.

I asked what he specifically recommends to build up resistance to the common cold. He advises: good diet, exercise, adequate rest and avoidance of stress. He further recommends the discovery and treatment of allergies, which will reduce the number of virus colds in an allergic individual.

In conclusion, he pointed out that allergens are usually proteins. It is the protein in foods, etc. to which people are sensitive. The protein in chocolate is irritating. Also an important final note was that chemicals in the air can give cold symptoms and that persistent allergies lead to sinus problems.

Interview with an Internist

In discussing questions with a leading California internist regarding the common cold and his treatment of it, I gathered the following information:

I learned that 10 percent of his patients come specifically to be treated for the common cold.

He pointed out that lower respiratory infection is lung

infection which is not a cold; neither is throat infection, alone, a cold.

With regard to treatment for nose and throat colds, he said if the patient's fever is over 101°, he prescribes antibiotics because fever indicates that the infection is usually bacterial in nature. For a runny nose, he prescribes nasal sprays and an antihistamine compound by mouth to shrink the mucous membrane. For a cough, he prescribes medication which contains something to suppress the cough and dry the mucous membrane. If the patient has a low fever—below 101°—he prescribes aspirin.

I asked him about bed rest, and he said he recommends it when possible, especially in severe cases.

With regard to my questions concerning vitamin C, fruit juices and supplements, he said he prescribes fruit juices because the body also needs fluids. He will prescribe supplements when the patient has an allergy to natural vitamin C.

When I asked if he eliminates anything specific from the diet, he said he does not.

I wondered what his thoughts were about smoking in relationship to a cold. He said if smoking irritates the patient, he will find out very quickly without the doctor's having to tell him.

To prevent reinfectivity, he recommends keeping away from crowds and especially from anyone with a cold.

I asked what he thinks the basic cause of most colds is. He answered, "Adenoviruses," (a virus partly responsible for the common cold).

Are dampness and cold important to the catching of the common cold, I asked. He answered that research has shown they are not, but, he added, he would have thought so if he hadn't learned the contrary through research.

He was especially interested in my question as to why children catch more colds than adults. He said that it could be due to more exposure to people in school and that children are more active and may play to the point of exhaustion. The doctor wants to give this problem more thought, as he realizes it is an important question.

In answer to my question, why are more colds caught in mid-winter than at any other time, he said there seems to be no season in California. He said there definitely is a cold season in cold countries, but it is not clear why.

In order to build up resistance to the common cold, he recommends: stay healthy, eat a balanced diet, get enough rest and have periodic medical checkups.

With regard to commercial cold remedies, he said that Coricidin is good; Contac can make one sick if taken too long without medical supervision; Dristan is helpful, but self-dosage is a bad idea. Vicks VapoRub, when applied to the chest, is of no value since there are many layers of tissue before the lungs are reached, and this medication cannot possibly penetrate the tissues or cross the air space to the lungs.

He concluded that most colds are caused by adenoviruses and some by bacteria. He pointed out that there is a vaccine for people who get one cold after another. It is called MVRI (Mixed Vaccine Respiratory Infection). However, he does not use it.

Interview with a Chiropractor

In discussing his care of the common cold with a Hollywood chiropractor, the following are his answers:

About 20 percent of his patients come to be treated specifically for the common cold.

His treatment for nose and throat colds is to give spinal adjustments to open blocked nerve channels. He pointed out that there are nine basic functions of life, controlled by the nervous system: reproductive, sensory, motor, calorific, nutritive, secretory, excretory, growth and repair. Each of these must be free of impingement in its nervous channels for the body to be healthy.

In answer to what is the main symptom he relies on in choosing a form of therapy, he said he checks the alignment of the atlas vertebra at the top of the spine because it is the first movable, physical link between the brain and the body.

With regard to bed rest, he recommends it depending on the severity of the cold as it allows the body to heal itself.

He recommends freshly squeezed orange or grapefruit juice. He does not recommend supplements, vitamins or mineral tablets.

With regard to eliminating anything specific from the diet, he said not to use anything canned, frozen or packaged. Use only natural foods. He recommends that one should fast during the cold.

"What do you recommend for a fever accompanying a cold?" I asked. He answered that one should fast and get proper vertebral correction so that the nervous system will oxidize the toxic effects of the cold through the normal eliminative channels.

To prevent reinfectivity, he advocates that one keep the nervous system clear of impingement so that the nine vital functions will keep up to par; also get proper nutrition (which he considers includes occasional fasts and fewer meats, eggs and heavy proteins. Actually, he recommends a total vegetarian diet if possible.)

He believes (as the basic cause) most colds are due to interference with one of the nine nerve channels—its function is impaired, throwing excess work onto the other channels.

He does not think that dampness and cold are important in the catching of a cold. They may, he said, trigger mechanisms that deflect the normal functions.

As to why children catch more colds than adults, his answer is, children fall more often, which upsets the nervous system. Another reason is that parents feed young infants too much canned baby food which has a built-up toxic effect. He believes that sometimes "cold" symptoms are merely an outgrowth of the changes and imbalances due to "growing" in a child.

With regard to more colds being caught in mid-winter, he felt it was due to weather change.

To build resistance to the common cold, he advocates the Grostic Method of spinal correction to make sure there is no pressure on nerves. Then next in importance is proper nutrition.

He does X rays from various angles of the neck and then does a mechanical analysis using geometric measurement to note displacement of spine.

In answer to my question regarding commercial cold remedies, he said they are detrimental to the system, that they treat the symptom without getting to the underlying cause.

Summation

Since my work is in the field of nutrition, I was particularly pleased to find one point on which the allergist, the internist and the chiropractor agreed—good nutrition as the way to build resistance against the common cold.

I deal with sound nutrition specifically in Chapters 18 and 20 and consider it of vital importance in the development of good health and prevention of the common cold.

17. Folk Cures, Folk Remedies and Superstitious Cures

Before the advent of modern relief for coryza (the common cold) almost every country—including our own—has used old folk cures for the common cold. Some of these are amazing, some amusing. These approaches to the common cold can be classified as folk cures, folk remedies and superstitous cures.

A folk cure is a homemade remedy which was and, in many cases, still is used by the inhabitants of a country to help cure a malady. It is handed down from generation to generation through the centuries. Folk remedies are also homemade measures, but they are used to *ease* the ill feeling brought on by a disease, they are not curative. They have been used throughout time whenever illness occurs. Superstitious cures are methods which are not based on reason or knowledge. They come out of a fear of the unknown, a belief in magic, in chance or the like.

167

Now, since we know something about the common cold, it can be fascinating to look back at some of the folk methods and superstitions for treating this illness.

The Chinese

The Chinese approached the cold in the following ways:
(1) They prescribed licorice to help subdue coughs due to colds.
(2) In ancient times Chinese farmers tried to cure the common cold by breathing the soothing vapors of a broomlike plant called "horse tail."

MY ANALYSIS

Modern-made licorice and all forms of flavored cough drops which contain white sugar are used today as a method of soothing an irritated throat. However, I disapprove of them, as they further irritate the throat, leading to reinfection. This is not an advisable way to ease the effects of a cold.

In regard to the "horse tail" vapors, the active ingredient was ephedrine—still widely used in nose sprays. This therapy was obviously a sound one, since the healing substance has stood the test of time. However, there are some doctors who will not prescribe it, as they claim it inhibits the action of the nasal cilia and is not considered curative.

Russia

The Russian farmers wrapped their hoarse throats in cloths containing a salted herring.

MY ANALYSIS

If nothing else, the aromatic fumes were enough to keep people away who had no colds, thereby cutting down on transmitting infection.

New Guinea

Inhabitants of the Papuan Gulf used large shields, painted with symbolic representations of ancestral spirits, to ward off illnesses associated with the common cold.

MY ANALYSIS

In uncivilized areas, the natives resorted to primitive methods. They knew no other way.

South America

In South America, the Araucanians and Chaco Indians performed ceremonies during which, after purifying themselves, they charged their invisible "cold enemies" and threatened them with their weapons.

MY ANALYSIS

Much like the aforementioned New Guinea inhabitants, the South American Indians believed that illnesses could be driven away like real foes.

Portugal

Onions are used in every form as a means of resisting and curing the common cold.

MY ANALYSIS

The curative element in raw onions is aldehydes, which are antiseptic.

France

In France they heated glass cups and placed them on a victim's back and chest to clear up congestion.

MY ANALYSIS

This is the old counter-irritation method used in the treatment of varying disorders. It is not advisable, since there is a risk of infection if the skin is abrased.

Other European Countries

(1) For centuries Europeans have eaten large quantities of garlic for the cure of the common cold. They believed that garlic held the cure for many an illness that would not respond to other remedies.

(2) Some Europeans in the seventeenth century treated colds by having patients put some of their hair between two slices of bread and then feed it to a dog.

MY ANALYSIS

(1) Dr. J. Klosa investigated why garlic could do what antibiotics and sulfa drugs had been unable to do. He reported his findings in the March, 1950, issue of a German magazine entitled *Medical Monthly*. Dr. Klosa found that garlic oil had an elusive ability to kill certain dangerous organisms without attacking the organisms vital to the body's health. Oil of garlic is composed, in part, of sulfides and disulfides. These unite with virus matter in such a way that the virus organisms are inactivated; consequently, their harmful effects cease, and they are prevented from any future activity. All this is done without any harm to healthful organisms in the body.

Dr. Klosa experimented with a solution of garlic oil and water, and he administered this preparation in doses of ten to twenty-five drops every four hours. It was found that the desired effect was enhanced by the inclusion of fresh extract of onion juice in the dosage.

(2) Perhaps they believed that the cold germs would be transferred to the dog.

Great Britain

An old and much-caricatured British remedy was to plant both feet firmly in a tub of hot water and sip some pacifying port.

An eighteenth century British physician proposed a popular form of therapy: "Hang your hat on a bedpost, drink from a bottle of good whiskey until two hats appear, then get into bed and stay there."

It is a known fact that warmth and rest are beneficial in bringing relief to a common cold sufferer. Any alcoholic beverage can bring temporary relief. However, it is not curative.

Eighty-six proof whiskey is more potent than the port and has about seven times more alcohol. This, too, is just temporary aid. Some doctors discourage the use of whiskey, as they claim it lowers the body's resistance. Others advocate it in moderation.

French Canada

The French Canadians used to treat bad colds by giving the victims molds growing on the tops of jams and jellies.

Whereas the molds might contain penicillin or some antibiotic, antibiotics are used primarily to fight bacterial infection. They are not used to combat virus infection which the cold is.

United States

(1) American colonials rinsed their nasal passages with sea water.

(2) Old-frontier cowboys crushed the leaves of wild thyme between their palms and inhaled the aromatic fumes.

(3) An old Texas cure for head colds and congestion consisted of wearing a necklace of onions and leeks for three successive days.

MY ANALYSIS

(1) Saline solutions are still used successfully as an anti-septic agent. For example, they are still prescribed today for a sore throat.

(2) Thyme is an herb, and it is a known fact that herbs have a curative effect.

(3) By the third day, presumably, everyone else had been driven from the house, and the sufferer could at least sneeze and wheeze away in peace and quiet.

As I review the cures, remedies and superstitious cures throughout time, it is very interesting to note how people helped themselves instinctively without the aid of medicine.

Part V
Nutrition

18. The Important Role of Sound Nutrition Introducing The Common Cold-Preventive Cocktail

What one eats is the barometer of one's health. A completely nutritive diet is essential not only to help prevent the common cold but practically all illnesses. For those who are already stricken with a cold, well-chosen foods, which I shall specify in Chapter 20, *will reduce the length of time the cold lasts* and possibly abort the cold within a day.

The respiratory tract is the seat of the common cold. In order for it to function well and ward off infection, proper nourishment is vital. The respiratory tract is made up of the nose, the sinuses, the throat, the nasopharynx, the larynx, the trachea and the bronchi leading down to the lungs. These organs can break down as a result of long-term malnutrition. This then makes one vulnerable not only to the common cold but to illnesses as serious as cancer. If the respiratory tract is to be maintained and sustained to its fullest potential, the body must receive sound nutrition. In Chapter 20, I recommend foods which will ensure the health of the respiratory system, and in Chapter 19, warn against foods which are harmful.

The right kind of nutrition is immediately reflected on the body. It supplies the essentials needed for the maintenance and functioning of the endocrine system. This system is composed of the thyroid (parathyroid), the adrenal glands, the pituitary, the thymus, the gonads (ovaries and testes), the pineal body and the pancreas. I want to stress the importance of the endocrine system, because it helps counteract any harmful attack on the body. When it functions normally, because of proper nutrition and consequent vitamins, a person's health is good, he sleeps well and, in general, he is able to perform productively in all aspects of his life. A further benefit is the production of better quality hormones which are essential for the health of the body. A healthy body will help resist the common cold.

Vitamins and Their Effectiveness

It has been pointed out, in articles dealing with the role of vitamins in relationship to the common cold, that vitamins A and D can help build resistance to disease, but they do not change the character of the blood. Henri Bourgeois, M.D., in an article in *Le Progrés Médical,* February 26, 1938, states that vitamin A produces only good results on the cells of the body tissue.

Lt. Col. J. Lavere Davidson, V.C., of the Sioux Falls, Army Air Field, reports in *Veterinary Medicine,* September,

1944, on how vitamin A works in the human body to prevent infection. He points out that the vitamin itself does not kill germs (for example cold or flu germs). Instead, "by direct action, vitamin A preserves the normal physiological functions and anatomical structure of the mucous membranes, and also aids in the regeneration and restoration of these membranes in the event they are injured or destroyed."

He further states that if a person does not have enough vitamin A in his diet, a change in the mucous membrane occurs. The cells with cilia slowly disappear and instead there will be hard, scaly cells which have no cilia. The secretions by the membranes are cut off and dryness results. Consequently, the cilia no longer sweep germs out of the respiratory passages, and the antiseptic secretions of the nose and throat no longer function. When a virus comes along, there is no defense against it.

Lt. Col. Davidson points out that vitamin A acts indirectly against colds, that it preserves the health and strength of the cells of the mucous membranes. Also, these cells are rejuvenated and replenished by vitamin A after they have been destroyed or injured by germs.

In Chapter 20, I give recommended menus with foods rich in vitamin A and a list of food supplements.

In the *British Medical Journal,* April 21, 1951, Drs. John M. and Isabel C. Fletcher state that, in treating their patients, they found vitamin C, when given in large quantities at the right time, to be an outstanding preventive of colds.

In an experiment with children in an institution in England, it was found that those who took vitamin C for six months were able, when they caught cold, to throw off the effects of their cold in half the time it took other afflicted children who did not take vitamin C.

W. J. McCormick, M.D., of Canada, in an article in the *Archives of Pediatrics,* reports that vitamin C in enormous doses is effective in curing disease. He points out that vitamin C is important for healing wounds, prevention of hemorrhaging and the building of resistance against germ invasion. It contributes to building antibodies in the bloodstream; it neutralizes toxins in the blood. It is instrumental in building a natural immunity to infectious diseases and poisons.

F. R. Klenner, M.D., of Reidsville, North Carolina, uses vitamin C with great success in treating his patients who have serious diseases. He reports, that in the case of a person suffering from a virus infection, vitamin C was absent in the urine and in the blood. The worse the infection gets, the more vitamin C is needed, since his body tissues are depleted, and whatever vitamin C he gets from his food is used up at once in trying to fight the virus. Therefore, Dr. Klenner gives massive doses of vitamin C when required.

Scientific researchers have found that bioflavonoids, a substance that appears in many fresh foods along with vitamin C, helps the body to use vitamin C properly. The two together are powerfully effective against the common cold.

In many articles, dealing with the common cold, massive doses of vitamin C are recommended to curb the infection. Bear in mind that no harm can come from such large amounts, as the excess is thrown off through the kidneys.

In London, in the summer of 1969, Nobel Laureate Dr. Linus Pauling advocated massive doses of vitamin C as a means of increasing protection against the common cold. He recommended, "Daily ingestion of 3000 to 6000 mg. of

ascorbic acid [as opposed to the usual 75 mg. a day] leads
to increased vigor, to increased protection against infectious
disease, including the common cold, and to an increased
rate of healing of wounds."

At this time I should like to emphasize the benefit of
natural vitamins as opposed to synthetic vitamins. Natural
vitamins are made from vitamins extracted from organic
foods grown in soil which has not been chemically treated.
They come in tablets, capsules and powders and can be
purchased primarily at health food stores. In my judgment
the synthetic vitamins are not as advantageous to the body as
natural vitamins.

A major reason natural vitamins are so beneficial is that
they contain enzymes. Enzymes are necessary for the proper
absorption of vitamins. There are no enzymes in synthetic
vitamins. New evidence indicates that both vitamins and

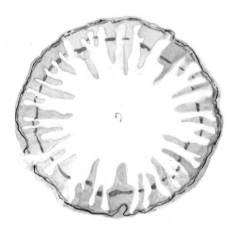

CHROMATOGRAM OF NATURAL VITAMIN B COMPLEX—NOTE OUTER
RIM: LONG, JAGGED TEETH INDICATE INTRINSIC FACTORS, GOOD PRO-
TEIN AND STRONG ENZYME ACTVITY.

trace minerals, to be beneficially effective, must be bound up in enzyme systems. This was pointed out by Dr. William P. McElroy, director of the McCullom Pratt Institute, Johns Hopkins University, before the National Academy of Science, Washington, D.C.

In 1953, Ehrenfried E. Pfeiffer, M.D., internationally known soil expert, perfected the Chromatogram for graphically demonstrating hidden differences in soils. He and his staff did their experimental work at their Biochemical Research Laboratory in Spring Valley, N.Y. He knew that frequently two soils might have almost the same chemical analysis but differ widely in biological values such as yield, quality of protein and seed germination. Through his use of pictures he could interpret qualitative and biological values.

Dr. Pfeiffer found he could also use Chromatograms to differentiate the values between two foods or two vitamins

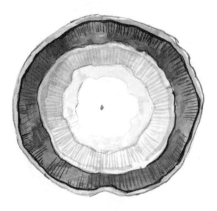

CHROMATOGRAM OF SYNTHETIC VITAMIN B COMPLEX—NOTE ABSENCE OF SPIKE-LIKE ENZYME FORMATIONS AND BIOLOGICAL INTRINSIC FACTORS.

which, though chemically identical, are widely different in biological and qualitative values. Every living thing has a purpose, and its juice displays a definite pattern in a Chromatogram. The fresher the product, the greater the biological activity and the more prominent the enzyme formations. The synthetic vitamin shows only colored rings but no definite pattern, for it is inert.

I present, herewith, two illustrations of Chromatograms to show the biological difference between synthetic vitamins and natural vitamins. The Chromatograms show that Nature does something that man cannot duplicate.

Vegetables, fruits, grains, dairy products and, to a lesser degree, meat, fowl and fish contain natural vitamins. I should like to point out that once these foods are cooked, the potency of the vitamins is very much diminished.

Foods grown in chemically treated soil do not yield the same high quality of vitamins. There is a difference!

Since vitamins play such an important role in building resistance against the common cold, I strongly recommend the use of natural vitamins because they are more effective. Some benefit can be derived from synthetic vitamins, but it is so slight that, in my opinion, there is little gained. If it is a case of taking synthetic vitamins or no vitamins at all, by all means take the synthetic vitamins.

Natural Body Defenses

To date there is no medication known that can kill the common cold virus. However, there are four natural body defenses that fight the common cold infection. They are the cilia, lysozyme, interferon and antibodies. In order to strengthen these, sound nutrition must be maintained.

Cilia and Mucous Membrane Nourishment

Sir Robert McCarrison, in the *Journal of the Royal Society of Arts,* September 4, 1936, points out that malnutrition can contribute to a condition in the nose that might create susceptibility to catching cold. He further states that the cilia (see Chapter 2) can perform their movements only when the membrane they fringe is moist and the moisture contains calcium. We can readily deduce from this the need for calcium in the diet in order to have well-functioning cilia and mucous membrane—*the first of the natural body defenses* that fight common cold virus infection.

As is generally known, milk is rich in calcium. Green vegetables and fresh fruit are also good sources of calcium. Bone meal or calcium tablets are concentrated doses of calcium and can be taken as supplements. Calcium benefits not only the cilia and mucous membrane but also the bones and teeth. Because vitamin D facilitates the proper assimilation of calcium, one should take one tablespoon of cod liver oil, which is rich in vitamin D, mixed with orange juice, on an empty stomach, in place of breakfast at least twice a month.

Some people have the mistaken notion that they are getting enough calcium for their body needs if they occasionally eat the milk products, cottage cheese or ice cream. However, it is necessary to have calcium in all three meals daily. Therefore, I strongly recommend drinking raw certified or homogenized milk with each meal as the best source for calcium. This will help build resistance against common cold virus infection.

Lysozyme Nourishment

The second natural body defense that fights common cold virus infection is lysozyme:

The secretion of the mucous glands not only work with the cilia to physically remove various objects, they also contain an enzyme, lysozyme. . . . Lysozyme was discovered and found to be a microbe-destroyer by Alexander Fleming (the discoverer of penicillin) in 1922. Since then, lysozyme has been shown to be active against viruses as well, as demonstrated by R. Ferrari and his colleagues in 1959 (*Nature* 183: 548). . . .

The two barriers we have described, however, depend on the health and efficient functioning of the mucous membrane. And this lining of the respiratory tract . . . deteriorates when it is not supplied with adequate vitamin A.[1]

It has been reported in *Interactions of Nutrition and Infection* that the activity of lysozyme "increased remarkably with five to seven days of cod-liver-oil therapy." Every ounce of cod-liver oil contains 1500 units of vitamin A and is, in my opinion, the most important source of vitamin A.

Interferon Nourishment

According to Sir Christopher Andrewes, in his book, *The Common Cold,* a possible mechanism for a nonspecific resistance to colds was brought to light by Dr. A. Isaacs in London and a Swiss collaborator, Dr. J. Lindenmann; this is

---

[1]*Prevention—The Magazine for Better Health,* February, 1970. Quoted by permission of Rodale Press, Inc.

interferon. In addition to the phenomenon of viral interference, whereby one virus interferes with the activity of another, even an unrelated one, there seems to be interference "mediated by a protein which has been called interferon. . . ."

It is produced by cells in quantity in response to certain stimuli, particularly the presence of dead or damaged virus. . . . If not disturbed a virus entering a cell causes the cell to stop its normal job and turn all its attention to making more virus instead. If the cell is, however, able to produce such interferon, the activities of the cell are switched by the presence of virus, and it goes on turning out interferon instead of virus. The virus-infection is halted. This is a mechanism of defense complementary to the production of neutralizing antibodies. It differs in three important respects. It is mobilized very quickly, a matter of hours instead of days. It is not specifically directed against the virus which elicits it, but acts against all sorts of viruses. On the other hand it is only effective over a relatively short period. This actually does not matter very much, as it has done its job by holding the fort until antibodies have had time to be produced. Interferon can be extracted from suitably stimulated cells, either in the whole animal or in tissue-culture and, at least in theory, can be applied to stop a virus infection. Numerous laboratory experiments hold out hope that this may be achieved, but so far interferon has not been produced in such quantity or in such a state of purity that it is practically effective. . . . Viruses differ in their sensitivity to interferon. Rhinoviruses appear to be amongst those which, in tissue culture at least, are most sensitive. . . .

It will be clear now that there is in interferon a possible mechanism for nonspecific protection against colds, whether they are due to rhinoviruses or other viruses. . . .

In an article entitled "Resistance and Immunity—A New Direction for Research," there is a very comprehensive section on interferon.[1] Because I found this to be the only material available which deals with my own concept of relating nutrition with interferon, I shall quote much of it:

> Another promising substance now getting a great deal of scientific attention is interferon, thought to be versatile enough to protect us from colds, flu, polio, smallpox and even cancer, yet so safe that side-effects need never be a problem. . . . Interferon . . . thought to be nature's universal vaccine against the insult of viral infections.
>
> When you say your resistance to diseases is good, what you mean is you are manufacturing sufficient interferon to fight off the viruses that cause colds, flu and a host of viral threats that are constantly blowing your way. . . .
>
> Science writer Fred Warshofsky tells us that Warren and Jensen and their associates working in a Pfizer laboratory in Terre Haute, Indiana, found that many nucleic acids would trigger animal cells into producing interferon. The nucleic acids are the basic chemical core of life, as well as the main components of viruses. Dozens of tests were made to find a nucleic acid inexpensive to produce, effective as a stimulator of interferon and harmless to the body cells. The final selection was the nucleic acid of a yeast (*True,* July, 1966).
>
> Perhaps when we consume food yeast which is rich in nucleic acid we are actually helping our bodies to kill offending viruses.

---

[1]*Prevention,* September, 1969. Quoted by permission of Rodale Press, Inc.

We could all feel more confident that our interferon is protecting us against virus invasions if it were not for a variety of obstacles created by our civilized environment. It has been found, for instance, that the carcinogens in our foods and environment exert a blocking effect on interferon production.

This was demonstrated by a husband and wife team of virologists, Edward and Jacqueline De Maeyer, who established a sinister connection between lack of interferon and the cancer-inducing compounds known as hydrocarbons. . . . There is a theory that people are constantly exposed to viruses capable of causing cancer. In the absence of outside agents such as hydrocarbons, the body shrugs off these viruses by increasing interferon production. But our increasing mechanization fills the air with hydrocarbons from auto exhausts, factory smoke and other sources; pesticides pollute our air and food supply with hydrocarbons; many of the residues in our foods are hydrocarbons. . . .

Air pollution is a chief cause of reduced interferon production, according to Dr. Samuel Baron of the Public Health Institute, Bethesda, Maryland. . . .

Cigarette smoking, long recognized as being related to the incidence of colds, is another inhibitor of interferon production and, according to Dr. Baron, most drugs will also interfere with the body's ability to produce interferon. This raises the distinct possibilty that every time you take a patent medicine to relieve a cold, you defeat your purpose, for you are, in effect, blocking the mechanism by which your body would cure the cold if you would only leave it alone.

If you give your body half a chance, you would be able to manufacture all the interferon you need to cure, or better yet, to prevent viral infections. Part of the answer obviously lies in those nutrients which help you to detoxify the chemical pollutants that are unavoidable in the air we breathe, the water we drink and the food we eat. Those of us who get enough vitamin C and B complex should be able to eliminate from our systems a large part of the toxic chemicals we are forced to take in every day. If we can get rid of them successfully and our cells are enjoying vigorous good health, our bodies will not be prevented from synthesizing the interferon we need to fight off a virus invasion.

Natural interferon is working for us all the time. Every healthy cell produces it as nature's way of keeping disease away. When researchers say the body is short of interferon, or resistance is low, they really mean that the body is short of cells healthy enough to produce their share. The key to producing enough interferon then is the key to keeping your cells healthy.

This knowledge simplifies the problem. We know how to keep a cell healthy. We know that our cells must have proper nutrition; that they must be able to withstand stress; that they cannot be constantly exposed to poisons. We know that if our cells are to be healthy our bodies must get sufficient rest. Also we must get an uninterrupted supply of oxygen. . . .

I presented my theory of sound nutrition as a means to help the body produce interferon to a leading virologist at a hospital in Los Angeles. He said that since interferon is thought to be a protein, though not yet purified, he believes that unless there is enough protein in the diet for making adequate amounts of all body proteins then it is unlikely the body can make interferon—*the third of the natural body defenses* that fight common cold virus infection.

Antibody Nourishment

According to Sir Christopher Andrewes, writing in *The Common Cold*:

> In response to injections of foreign proteins or to invasion by bacteria or viruses, the body produces antibodies. These are modified forms of protein circulating in the blood and they combine with the foreign protein or microbe to render it harmless. The chemical substance which stimulates formation of an antibody is called an antigen. Two viruses or other microbes which differ in their chemical make-up elicit correspondingly different antibodies and are said to differ antigenically. . . . The antibodies may neutralize or inactivate a virus so that it no longer produces a disease in an inoculated animal nor leads to changes in an infected tissue culture; or the antibody may form a visible precipitate when mixed with the corresponding antigen; or the antibody may inhibit the clumping by virus of red blood cells. . . .

The leading virologist at a hospital in Los Angeles, to whom I presented my theory of sound nutrition as a means to help the body produce natural defenses against the common cold, indicated that since antibodies are protein, here too, unless there is enough protein in the diet for making adequate amounts of all body proteins, it is unlikely the body can make antibodies—the *fourth of the natural body defenses* that fight common cold virus infection.

I have already pointed out in this chapter (in the section "Vitamins and Their Effectiveness") the necessity of vitamins to help build up antibodies. In Chapter 20, I give menus which will also aid the production of antibodies.

The Common Cold-Preventive Cocktail

I shall now, for the first time, introduce my Common Cold-Preventive Cocktail—*a new way of eating* which will effectively and quickly build resistance to the common cold. This is a new concept which I have conceived. I have experimented with this myself and with many others and have found it to be:

(1) Helpful in preventing a cold.

(2) Helpful in reducing the time of a cold

(3) Helpful in some cases in aborting a cold within a day

The Common Cold-Preventive Cocktail is a potent liquid breakfast. It is composed of many nutrients, most of which can be digested and assimilated within the short period of one hour. The advantage of this rapid assimilation is that there is almost instantaneous nourishment which strengthens the body's natural defenses in their fight against infection. Starting the day with this highly nutritious meal, followed by lunch and dinner according to the menus in Chapter 20, is an assured way to acquire better health, tremendous energy and resistance to the common cold.

Some of the elements necessary to help the body produce the four natural body defenses (the cilia, lysozyme, interferon and antibodies) against the common cold have already been indicated earlier in this chapter. The Common Cold-Preventive Cocktail contains not only all of these ingredients but others as well.

The recipe will be given at the end of this chapter. If it

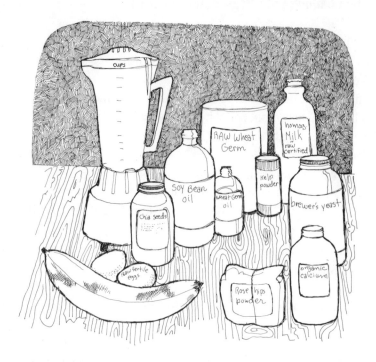

THE COMMON COLD-PREVENTIVE COCKTAIL—NEW, EFFECTIVE, QUICK WAY TO HELP PREVENT A COLD, HELP REDUCE TIME OF A COLD AND HELP ABORT A COLD WITHIN A DAY.

is prepared according to directions and drunk on an empty stomach every morning as a complete breakfast (be sure nothing is eaten until lunch) *the entire body will be thoroughly nourished* which will ensure resistance against the common cold.

I shall list below what the cocktail contains to strengthen

the body as a whole and to help produce the four natural body defenses:

(1) To ensure a well-functioning respiratory tract, the cocktail contains calcium, B complex and vitamin A.

(2) To ensure a well-functioning endocrine system, the cocktail contains vitamins B, D and organic iodine.

(3) To ensure well-functioning mucous membrane and cilia, the cocktail contains vitamin A and calcium.

(4) To help the body produce lysozyme, the cocktail contains vitamin B.

(5) To help the body produce interferon, the cocktail contains nucleic acid, vitamins C, B complex and protein.

(6) To help the body produce antibodies, the cocktail contains vitamins B, C and protein.

(7) In addition, the cocktail contains raw minerals, raw carbohydrates, raw hormones and raw enzymes.

Recipe for the Common Cold-Preventive Cocktail

Into a blender put the following ingredients:

2 cups raw certified or homogenized milk
4 raw eggs, preferably fertile

Turn on the motor. Then add:

2 teaspoons wheat germ oil
2 teaspoons either soybean or safflower oil

2 teaspoons powdered organic calcium
   or bone meal powder
1 tablespoon brewer's yeast
½ teaspoon kelp powder
2 teaspoons rose hips powder
4 tablespoons raw wheat germ
1 teaspoon chia seeds

If the mixture is thicker than you desire, add more milk.

1 ripe banana

Let the motor run an additional minute.

This will make approximately one quart. It should be refrigerated immediately and can be kept for up to six days.

Drink one 10-oz. glassful of this cocktail on an empty stomach for your complete breakfast.

If you have an overweight problem, drink 6 oz.

If you are underweight or do hard physical work, drink two 10-oz. glassfuls of the cocktail.

Note: Chia seeds have gelatin in them. When they are dissolved, they will thicken the cocktail. Therefore, be sure you do not put them in until prior to the fruit as listed.

You may want to use other fruits occasionally in place of the ripe banana. Choose any one of the following:

½ papaya
½ apple
12 boysenberries
12 cranberries

The ingredients for the cocktail can be purchased in health food stores. Whatever they don't have in stock they will order for you. If there is no health food store in your area, you can find one in a larger nearby city. They will ship your order to you if you write or phone them. There are supermarkets which carry some of these items.

I want to emphasize that the total effect of this cocktail will be *almost instantly increased health* which will mean *almost immediate resistance to the common cold,* because all the natural body defenses will be strengthened.

19. Harmful Beverages, Foods and Eating Habits, With Exceptions

It is extremely important to avoid harmful beverages and foods as they can impair one's health and thereby lower resistance to the common cold and other diseases. Such eating mistakes can negate the benefits that can be gained from the Common Cold-Preventive Cocktail and the nutritive foods I recommend in Chapter 20. Let me assure you that the regimen I suggest contains all the necessary nutrients and will also replace the minimal amount that may be in the beverages and foods I shall urge you to avoid.

It is also imperative to avoid eating habits—ways of drinking and eating—which are harmful. The average person usually confuses harmful eating habits with harmful foods. I shall present what I believe to be harmful eating habits. They consist of what I call "Wrong Timing in Drinking Oil-free

Liquids with Solid Foods," "Wrong Temperature of Liquids," and "The Wrong Preparation of Food." This information will be interspersed in the subsequent material dealing with harmful beverages and foods.

Harmful Beverages and the Wrong Timing in Drinking Oil-free Liquids with Solid Foods

I have observed that the grave mistake most people make is to drink either water, coffee, tea, soft drinks, frozen fruit juices, vegetable juices, beer, alcoholic drinks or other oil-free liquids with their meals. To use ice cubes in any of these drinks with meals makes it even more hazardous.

It is harmful to drink any of these liquids with meals because it prevents the dietary oils in the solid foods from being properly assimilated. Proper assimilation of food is vital to one's health.

I want to emphasize that the *Wrong Timing in Drinking Oil-Free Liquids with Solid Foods* is a harmful eating habit which must be avoided. The above mentioned beverages *must not be drunk with meals*.

Permissible Beverages

Oil-free beverages such as water, herb tea, fresh carrot and tomato juices, freshly squeezed orange juice including the pulp can be drunk approximately 10 minutes before or 4 hours after the meal.

Wrong Temperature of Liquids

I am thoroughly opposed to iced drinks, because they prevent proper assimilation, accelerate the heartbeat, and elevate the blood cholesterol. However, if you must have them, do not drink them with food. They should only be drunk on an empty stomach 10 minutes before or 6 hours after a meal.

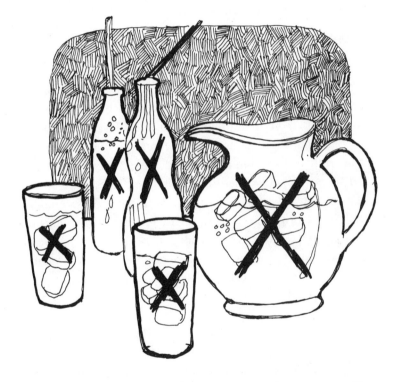

WRONG TEMPERATURE OF LIQUIDS—DO NOT DRINK ICED DRINKS WITH MEALS, AS THEY WILL PREVENT PROPER ASSIMILATION, ACCELERATE HEARTBEAT AND ELEVATE THE BLOOD CHOLESTEROL.

Recommended Liquids with Meals

I strongly recommend that you drink milk with each solid meal and soup with either lunch or dinner. *These are the only liquids permissible with meals.* They are compatible with the dietary oils in the solid foods as they contain oil and have low surface tension.

Juices

Fruit juices, such as grapefruit, lemon, boysenberry, raspberry, papaya, guava and prune, and vegetable juices, such as celery, should be drunk only occasionally because the cellulose and other vital nutrients are usually lost in the process of being liquified. Therefore, it is preferable to eat these foods whole rather than liquified. When these foods are eaten in solid form, the saliva neutralizes any acid they may contain.

From many years of observation, I have discovered that people who drink large amounts of grapefruit, lemon, grape and pineapple juices, over a long period of time, have dry skin, dermatitis, psoriasis, bad breath and get prematurely gray or white hair. Overall they have poor health which means lowered resistance and susceptibility to the common cold.

The reason for these disorders is that grapefruit, lemon, grape and pineapple juices contain more acid than the saliva. Because of this, when these juices are consumed, the body is forced to use buffer salts which have to be taken from the skin and other tissues in order to neutralize this excessive acidity. This results in the harmful effects mentioned above.

The Destructive Carbonated Soft Drink

The most destructive beverage is the soft drink because it contains white sugar, carbonated gas and phosphoric acid. Since the danger of cyclamates has been recognized they are no longer used in drinks. White sugar robs the body of B vitamins. Carbonated gas finds its way to the weakest organs in the body and does further damage to them. It makes one prone to peptic and duodenal ulcers. Scientists have found that phosphoric acid induces cancer in experimental animals.

It is harmful to mix any alcoholic beverages with soda, colas, ginger ale, tonic or any other mixes because they are gaseous liquids which harm the body. I personally am opposed to all alcoholic beverages. However, if you wish to have occasional drinks, drink them straight or with water ten minutes or more before and four to six hours after meals.

Avoid Chocolate Milk

I have already pointed out in a previous chapter that commercially made chocolate milk or the homemade preparation which is sticky chocolate syrup added to milk and not thoroughly blended are harmful and will make one vulnerable to the common cold.

To sum up, avoid the beverages that are harmful in themselves or when drunk at the wrong time.

Foods That Harm the Respiratory Tract

It has been found that too much and the wrong kind of carbohydrate in the diet is apparently closely related to colds and other troubles of the respiratory tract.

Foods that harm the respiratory tract and should be avoided are white sugar, pastry, processed cereals and processed wheat flour products such as bread, cakes, doughnuts, pies, macaroni and spaghetti. Refined wheat products, in particular, affect the nasal mucus which can be associated with the onset of a cold.

Dr. E. Seaver, Jr., in an article in the *Transactions of the American Laryngology, Rhinology and Otolaryngy Society,* vol. 44, makes an excellent analysis of why refined carbohydrates have a bad effect on throat, nasal and sinus passages. He states it is generally accepted by nutrition experts that a diet high in refined carbohydrates (white sugar and white flour products) is automatically low in minerals and vitamins as well as cellulose which is needed to assure the proper working of one's digestive tract. If you eat a highly refined carbohydrate diet, your need for B vitamins is automatically increased.

It, therefore, is important to recognize that because highly refined carbohydrates are harmful to the respiratory tract they lower resistance to the common cold. However, the foods that actually trigger the common cold are chocolate products, caramel, frosting, jelly and any other sticky sweets added to bakery, candy products or desserts.

A further risk in long-term consumption of highly refined carbohydrates is that it can lead to the development of allergies.

Natural Carbohydrates

Do not confuse natural carbohydrates, which are nutritious, with refined carbohydrates, which are harmful. The natural carbohydrates are fresh fruits, fresh vegetables and whole-grain cereals. It is preferable to eat these foods in their natural state because, as such, they are more powerful in building resistance. If cooked, there is some value, though to a far lesser degree.

Foods That Rob the Body

There are foods that actually rob the body of vitamins. Foods made from white flour and white sugar have had their own vitamin B removed, and they in turn rob the body of its vitamin B. Therefore, as already pointed out, these must be avoided.

Avoid Salt

Egon V. Ullmann, M.D., in his book, *Diet in Sinus Infection and Colds* (New York, Macmillan Company), advises a salt-poor diet for chronic cold sufferers. The sodium part of table salt is what he warns against. Sodium cancels out the excellent and necessary functions of calcium. With a reduction of sodium chloride in the diet, the calcium action will prevail and lead up toward an anti-inflammatory effect.

In April, 1970, an article was published in the *Proceedings of the Society for Experimental Biology and Medicine,* which set forth the newest evidence that common salt in commercial baby food may lead to high blood pressure in later life in babies genetically prone to the disease.

Dr. Lewis K. Dahl, senior scientist and chief of staff at Brookhaven's Research Hospital, urged that food processors make foods without added salt, and that mothers feed their babies foods without added salt.

It is a well-established fact that excessive use of table salt constricts arteries. I am concerned particularly with well-functioning kidneys as a cold-sufferer must have good elimination in order to hasten recovery. If he avoids salt this will help. Another reason to avoid salt is that constricted arteries cause the heart to work harder. This can lead to damage to the heart.

Acid-Forming Foods

Egon V. Ullman, M.D., in *Diet in Sinus Infections and Colds,* points out that proteins are important to a good diet and that it is very difficult to get enough good, first-class protein without the animal foods—milk, meat, fish and eggs. However, it is well to remember that these foods are acid-forming in the body and must be balanced with foods that have alkaline reaction. These are, in general, the fruits and vegetables.

There is one other group of foods—the cereals—that form acid in the body. In the United States, other foods made almost entirely of refined, white, wheat flour are bread, toast, crackers, biscuits, rolls, buns, doughnuts, cakes, pies, puddings, waffles, wafers, etc. If eaten, the consequences are lack of calcium and valuable minerals, a tendency toward acidosis, poor teeth, gas, constipation and sluggishness, according to Dr. Ullmann.

He advocates that sufferers from colds and sinusitis should eat rye bread, graham bread and pumpernickel whenever possible. All cereals should be unrefined. Sugar should be omitted entirely from diet to help avoid colds and sinusitis.

The Wrong Preparation of Food

The third harmful eating habit to be avoided is "The Wrong Preparation of Food" which I shall describe below:

(1) Do not peel the skin off of vegetables and fruits, as it is a rich source of minerals and vitamins.

(2) It is far more nutritious for vegetables and fruit *not to be cooked,* as the enzyme, mineral and vitamin contents will not be dissipated. However, cooked vegetables and fruits have some nutritive value.

(3) The skin of fish and fowl should not be trimmed off, because it contains essential nutrients.

(4) Fat should be trimmed from meats, as, if it is consumed along with oil-free liquids, it increases the manufacture of cholesterol in the body.

(5) Food should not be fried, because when oil is heated to a high temperature it cannot be properly assimilated.

Sample Meals Which Cause Common Cold Vulnerability

A WRONG BREAKFAST
FOR ADULTS

Frozen orange juice
Processed cereal
White bread toast and jelly
Frosted sweet roll
Black coffee with sugar

A WRONG BREAKFAST
FOR CHLDREN

Frozen orange juice
Sugar-coated dry cereal
Glazed doughnuts
Homemade chocolate milk
RECESS: *Frosted cupcake*

A WRONG LUNCH
FOR ADULTS

Macaroni
Glass of iced water
Chocolate meringue pie
Cola drink

A WRONG LUNCH
FOR CHILDREN

Macaroni
Chocolate-covered cookies
Homemade chocolate milk
AFTER SCHOOL
Bar of chocolate candy

A WRONG DINNER
FOR ADULTS

Iced vodka and tonic
Spaghetti
Chocolate layer cake
Black coffee with sugar

A WRONG DINNER
FOR CHILDREN

Iced water
Spaghetti
White bread
Hot fudge sundae
TV SNACK: *Assorted candies*

The sample meals contain foods which are unfortunately eaten by many children and adults. Were they questioned with regard to the incidence of colds contracted, I am certain they would admit to being cold victims many times a year.

I have already pointed out in the early part of this chapter that the foods and liquids listed in the sample meals are harmful. Some cause a lowering of resistance to the common cold, and others—the chocolate and other sticky sweets— actually trigger and cause the common cold, *if eaten in the presence of a common cold carrier.*

I strongly urge, even though these foods and the others I have warned against may be among your favorites, *eliminate them for all time from your diet.* This sacrifice will bring the reward of health and no colds.

20. Menus: Nourishing Foods Which Help Build Resistance Against the Common Cold

My effective, proven, common cold-resistance-building *new way of eating* is made up of *one liquid meal*—the Common Cold-Preventive Cocktail, described in Chapter 18—and *two solid meals* daily. After careful and extensive experimentation with combinations of solid foods, I can now present lunch and dinner menus which will further ensure good health, help build resistance to the common cold, and, if you are stricken, reduce the length of time the cold lasts and possibly abort the cold within a day.

207

The Alexander Vegetable Salad

The Alexander Vegetable Salad contains prime nutrients, rich in minerals and vitamins. This tossed salad is far more nutritious than the ordinary vegetable salad usually served with various dressings.

My salad is constructed mostly with sets of two to three vegetables at a time, then tossed each time with highly nutritive herbs, seeds, fruit concentrate powders and raw nuts. Preparing the salad in this way results in an even distribution of exotic flavors throughout. Every bite is uniform in taste.

If any salad is left over, it can be used for days thereafter, since the lemon juice, enzyme seasonings and lemon concentrate powder keep it fresh and tasty.

Recipe for the Alexander Vegetable Salad

INGREDIENTS

1 bunch green parsley
1 bunch green watercress
2 heads of romaine lettuce
6 green onions, including shoots (scallions)
1 large red sweet onion
1 4-oz. bag greenish alfalfa sprouts
3 medium-size beige Jerusalem artichokes
1 green or red pepper
2 raw ears of yellow sweet corn
2 large red tomatoes

SEASONINGS
> **9 tablespoons of either sunflower seed
>   oil, safflower or soybean oil**
> **½ teaspoon hickory smoked enzyme
>   seasoning**
> **½ teaspoon oregano**
> **1 teaspoon lemon concentrate powder**
> **1 teaspoon orange concentrate powder**
> **½ teaspoon organic mineral powder**
> **4 tablespoons apple cider vinegar**
> **2 tablespoons fresh lemon juice**
> **6 tablespoons almond meal**

All of these items can be bought in most health food stores. In some cases, supermarkets will take orders for them. If you are unable to get all of the seasonings, use whatever is available.

DIRECTIONS

Wash and drain all vegetables. Do not remove the skin of any of the vegetables except of the red onion and sweet corn.

Cut up the parsley and watercress into ¼-inch pieces.

Tear up the 2 heads of romaine lettuce into ½-inch pieces.

Coat a large, wooden salad bowl with 3 tablespoons of oil.

Put the parsley, watercress and romaine lettuce in the salad bowl.

Toss until all the vegetables are covered with oil.

Sprinkle the parsley, watercress and romaine lettuce with a portion of:
>   hickory smoked enzyme seasoning

oregano
lemon concentrate powder
orange concentrate powder
Toss.

Note that the seasonings cling to the oil-coated vegetables.

Dice 6 green onions and the red onion. Add to the salad.
Toss.

Sprinkle all the vegetables with another portion of:
hickory smoked enzyme seasoning
oregano
lemon concentrate powder
orange concentrate powder
Toss.

Sprinkle the salad with ¼ teaspoon of organic mineral powder. Pour 2 tablespoons of apple cider vinegar and 1 tablespoon of fresh lemon juice over the salad.
Toss.

Mix all the alfalfa sprouts into the salad. Cut the Jerusalem artichokes into slivers. Add to the salad.
Toss.

Dice the green or red pepper. Slice off the kernels of the raw sweet corn. Add to the salad. Sprinkle the salad with 3 tablespoons of almond meal.
Toss.

Add the remaining 6 tablespoons of oil to the salad.
Toss.

Add the remaining:
>   hickory smoked enzyme seasoning
>   oregano
>   lemon concentrate powder
>   orange concentrate powder
>   organic mineral powder
>   *Toss.*

Cut up the 2 tomatoes into ⅛s and put into the salad. Toss lightly to protect the tomatoes from being crushed.

Add remaining lemon juice and apple cider vinegar.
>   *Toss.*

Sprinkle the remaining almond meal on the top of the salad. The salad is ready to serve. If you wish, chill it.

For variation you may add cooked, fresh shrimp, lobster, crab meat, tuna fish, diced cheddar cheese, diced chicken, pieces of cold roast beef or any leftover meats. Add mayonnaise to taste. Toss for the final time. This salad makes six to eight generous servings.

The Alexander Fruit Salad

The Alexander Fruit Salad contains prime nutrients, rich in natural carbohydrates, minerals, vitamins, enzymes, pectin and bioflavonoids.

My salad is constructed with mostly sets of two to three fruits at a time, coated with yogurt and tossed with highly nutritive fruit concentrate powders and almond nut meal. As a consequence, there is an even distribution of exotic flavors throughout the salad. Every bite is uniform in taste.

If any salad is left over, it can be used for days thereafter since the lemon juice, enzyme seasoning and fruit concentrate powders keep it fresh and tasty.

Recipe for the Alexander Fruit Salad

INGREDIENTS
(IF POSSIBLE USE
ORGANICALLY GROWN FRUIT)

3 red delicious apples
3 green pippin apples
3 oranges
1 pink grapefruit
1 ripe cantaloupe
½ lb. red Tokay grapes
½ lb. blue ribonier grapes
1 fresh pineapple
3 ripe bananas

SEASONINGS

1 pint plain yogurt
1 tablespoon lemon concentrate powder
1 tablespoon orange concentrate powder
4 tablespoons fresh lemon juice
8 tablespoons almond meal
6 tablespoons malted coconut powder

All of these items can be bought in most health food stores. In some cases, supermarkets will take orders for them. If you are unable to get all of the seasonings, use whatever is available.

DIRECTIONS

Wash and drain the fruit. Leave the skin on the apples.

Coat a large, wooden salad bowl with ½ pint of plain yogurt.

Cut apples into ¼ s, and then cut each piece in half crosswise. Put into salad bowl.

Toss until fruit is covered with yogurt.

Peel oranges and grapefruit. Separate into sections. Cut each section in half crosswise. Put into salad bowl.
 Toss.

Sprinkle ½ of the lemon concentrate powder, ½ of the orange concentrate powder and ½ of the malted coconut powder on the fruit. Add ½ of the lemon juice. Sprinkle ½ of the almond meal on the salad.
 Toss.

The seasonings will cling to each piece of fruit.
Skin and dice the cantaloupe. Put into salad.
 Toss.

Remove the stems from the red and blue grapes. Put the grapes into the salad.
 Toss.

Peel and dice the pineapple. Put into the salad.
 Toss.

Add remaining yogurt.
> *Toss.*

Add the balance of the lemon concentrate powder, the orange concentrate powder and the malted coconut powder. Slice the bananas, after peeling, and put into the salad.

Toss lightly to avoid crushing the bananas.

Sprinkle the balance of the almond meal over the top of the salad.
> *Do not toss.*

Cover and chill. This salad makes six to eight generous servings.

The Menus

Herewith are three sets of menus, designed for normal-weight, underweight and overweight people. You will note that the foods listed are relatively the same but differ in quantities. These are suggested, sample menus to follow. However, for variety, you may select foods from the master list at the end of this chapter. Bear in mind, when making substitutions to keep the quantities consistent with the originally planned menus.

Seven Days of Menus for Those with Normal Weight

Monday

BREAKFAST:

*Common Cold-Preventive Cocktail
    (1 10-oz. glass, blended and taken as
    described in Chapter 18)*

LUNCH:

*Alexander Vegetable Salad
    (medium portion)
Broiled lean hamburger on wheat roll
    (8 oz.)
Milk (8-oz. glass)*

DINNER:

*Homemade soup (1 bowl)
Broiled steak (8 oz.)
Alexander Vegetable Salad
    (medium portion)
Fresh fruit
Milk (8-oz. glass)*

Tuesday

BREAKFAST:

*Common Cold-Preventive Cocktail
    (1 10-oz. glass)*

LUNCH:

Tuna fish sandwich on whole wheat toast
Alexander Fruit Salad
  (medium portion)
Milk (8-oz. glass)

DINNER:

Consommé (1 cup)
Broiled liver steak (8 oz.)
Steamed onions (½ cup)
Brown rice (½ cup)
Green celery and carrot sticks
Wedge of cheese
Milk (8-oz. glass)

Wednesday

BREAKFAST:

Common Cold-Preventive Cocktail
  (1 10-oz. glass)

LUNCH:

Vegetable soup (1 bowl)
Broiled cheeseburger on toasted wheat
  roll (8 oz.)
Raw red onion (1 slice)
Milk (8-oz. glass)

DINNER:

Alexander Vegetable Salad (medium portion)

Broiled salmon steak (6 oz.)
Baked potato with sour cream and chives
Strawberries and cream (or other berries
*   in season)*
Milk (8-oz. glass)

Thursday

BREAKFAST:

Common Cold-Preventive Cocktail
*   (1 10-oz. glass)*

LUNCH:

Whole wheat crackers and cheese
Mushroom and barley soup (1 bowl)
Fresh fruit
Milk (8-oz. glass)

DINNER:

Broiled hamburger (8 oz.)
Raw red onion (1 slice)
Baked potato with sweet butter
Apple
Raw, unsalted almonds (¼ cup)
Milk (8-oz. glass)

Friday

BREAKFAST:

Common Cold-Preventive Cocktail
*   (1 10-oz. glass)*

LUNCH:

Tomato and rice soup (1 bowl)
Rye crackers and sweet butter
Banana and apple salad with shredded
  coconut (medium portion)
Milk (8-oz. glass)

DINNER:

Alexander Vegetable Salad
  (medium portion)
Broiled halibut (8 oz.)
Brown rice (½ cup)
Fresh fruit
Raw, unsalted cashews (¼ cup)
Milk (8-oz. glass)

Saturday

BREAKFAST:

Common Cold-Preventive Cocktail
  (1 10-oz. glass)

LUNCH:

Organic hot dogs (2)
  (from health food store)
Homemade baked beans
  (no molasses)
  (1 cup)
Fresh pineapple wedges

Plain yogurt (8 oz.)
Milk (8-oz. glass)

DINNER:

Alexander Vegetable Salad
*   (medium portion)*
Lean roast beef (8 oz.)
Baked potato with sour cream and chives
Raw, unsalted pecan nuts (¼ cup)
Milk (8-oz. glass)

Sunday

BREAKFAST:

Common Cold-Preventive Cocktail
*   (1 10-oz. glass)*

LUNCH:

Lentil soup (1 bowl)
Wheat crackers
Cottage cheese (1 cup) with cantaloupe
Milk (8-oz. glass)

DINNER:

Alexander Vegetable Salad
*   (medium portion)*
Broiled chicken (½ chicken)
Brown rice (½ cup)
Raisins (½ cup)
Raw, unsalted filberts (¼ cup)
Milk (8-oz. glass)

Suggestions to Underweight People

(1) Eat larger portions of food than you have been eating.

(2) Eat generous portions of pumpkin and sunflower seeds as often as possible.

(3) Cod Liver Oil Mixture: make a mixture of 1 tablespoon of cod liver oil and 4 oz. of milk. Shake well in a small screw-top jar. Drink before retiring, approximately 4 hours after the evening meal. Take every night for 6 months, thereafter once a week.

(4) Take 1 tablespoon of wheat germ oil 3 times a week during the afternoon.

(5) Use generous portions of butter.

(6) If for any reason you cannot take the Common Cold-Preventive Cocktail, eat both whole grain cereal and eggs for breakfast.

(7) Eliminate all coffee and ordinary tea. (I recommend only *herb* teas, to be drunk on an empty stomach.)

(8) Eat soup as often as you can, especially lentil, bean, and mushroom and barley soups.

(9) Eat generous amounts of raw, unsalted almonds, cashews, Brazil nuts, pecans, filberts and walnuts.

(10) Drink a glass of milk 1 hour after your evening meal. If you carry out the above suggestions and eat the following meals, you will gain weight and help build resistance to the common cold.

Seven Days of Menus for Those Who are Underweight

Monday

BREAKFAST:

*Common Cold-Preventive Cocktail
(2 10-oz. glasses, blended and taken as
described in Chapter 18.)*

LUNCH:

*Lentil soup (1 bowl)
Grilled cheese sandwich (whole grain
bread)
Alexander Vegetable Salad
(large portion)
Milk (10-oz. glass)*

4:00 P.M.

Pumpkin seeds (½ cup)

DINNER:

*Broiled chicken (½ chicken)
Baked potato with butter
Green celery (4 stalks)
Alexander Fruit Salad (large portion)
Milk (10-oz. glass)*

1 HOUR LATER:

*Milk (10-oz. glass)
Sunflower seeds (¼ cup)*

BEFORE RETIRING:

Cod Liver Oil Mixture
   (See suggestion 3 above.)

Tuesday

BREAKFAST:

Common Cold-Preventive Cocktail
   (2 10-oz. glasses)

LUNCH:

Mushroom and barley soup (1 bowl)
Whole grain buttered toast (2 slices)
Tuna fish salad (large portion)
Tomato and cucumber slices with romaine
   lettuce—Roquefort dressing
1 Banana with cream
Milk (10-oz. glass)

4:00 P.M.

1 tablespoon wheat germ oil

DINNER:

Alexander Vegetable Salad
   (large portion)
Broiled liver and onions (8 oz.)
Baked potato with sour cream and chives
Alexander Fruit Salad
   (large portion)
Milk (10-oz. glass)

1 HOUR LATER:

Milk (10-oz. glass)

BEFORE RETIRING:

Cod Liver Oil Mixture

Wednesday

BREAKFAST:

*Common Cold-Preventive Cocktail
  (2 10-oz. glasses)*

LUNCH:

*Navy bean soup (1 bowl)
Roast beef sandwich (whole wheat bread)
Carrot and raisin salad
1 Banana with cream
Milk (10-oz. glass)*

4:00 P.M.

Pumpkin seeds (½ cup)

DINNER:

*Shrimp cocktail
Broiled lobster or fish of choice
Baked potato with butter
Alexander Vegetable Salad
  (large portion)
Melon (in season)
Milk (10-oz. glass)*

1 HOUR LATER:

Milk (10-oz. glass)

BEFORE RETIRING:

Cod Liver Oil Mixture

Thursday

BREAKFAST:

Common Cold-Preventive Cocktail
   (2 10-oz. glasses)

LUNCH:

Cream cheese and raisin sandwich
   (whole grain bread)
Alexander Fruit Salad
   (with whipped cream)
Raw, unsalted mixed nuts (½ cup)
Milk (10-oz. glass)

4:00 P.M.

1 tablespoon wheat germ oil

DINNER:

Barley and bean soup (1 bowl)
Broiled steak (12 oz.)
Steamed brown rice (1 cup)
   (with butter)
Alexander Vegetable Salad (large portion)

*1 Banana, blueberries and yogurt with
   shredded coconut*
Milk (10-oz. glass)

1 HOUR LATER:

Milk (10-oz. glass)

BEFORE RETIRING:

Cod Liver Oil Mixture

Friday

BREAKFAST:

*Common Cold-Preventive Cocktail
   (2 10-oz. glasses)*

LUNCH:

Crabmeat cocktail
Split pea soup (1 bowl)
Broiled hamburger (12 oz.)
*Alexander Vegetable Salad
   (large portion)*
Milk (10-oz. glass)

4:00 P.M.

*Mixed raw, unsalted nuts with Black
   Monukka raisins (½ cup)*

DINNER:

Alexander Vegetable Salad (large portion)

Broiled salmon steak (12 oz.)
Baked potato with butter
Melon (in season)
Yogurt and sliced banana
Milk (10-oz. glass)

1 HOUR LATER:

Milk (10-oz. glass)

BEFORE RETIRING:
Cod Liver Oil Mixture

Saturday

BREAKFAST:

Common Cold-Preventive Cocktail
   (2 10-oz. glasses)

LUNCH:

Lentil soup (1 bowl)
Organic hot dogs (2)
   (from health food store)
Toasted whole grain bun
Baked beans (no molasses)
Cole slaw (½ cup)
Mixed raw, unsalted nuts (½ cup)
Milk (10-oz. glass)

4:00 P.M.

1 tablespoon wheat germ oil

DINNER:

Alexander Vegetable Salad
  (large portion)
Roast beef (12 oz.)
Baked potato with sour cream and chives
Alexander Fruit Salad (large portion)
Milk (10-oz. glass)

1 HOUR LATER:

Milk (10-oz. glass)

BEFORE RETIRING:

Cod Liver Oil Mixture

Sunday

BREAKFAST:

Common Cold-Preventive Cocktail
  (2 10-oz. glasses)

LUNCH:

Lima bean soup (1 bowl)
Cottage cheese, berries and sour cream
Cold meat sandwich (whole grain bread)
1 Banana
Milk (10-oz. glass)

4:00 P.M.

Mixture of sunflower and pumpkin seeds
  (½ cup)

DINNER:

Alexander Vegetable Salad
   (large portion)
Broiled steak (12 oz.)
Baked potato with butter
Steamed brown rice (½ cup)
Alexander Fruit Salad
   (large portion)
Milk (10-oz. glass)

1 HOUR LATER:

Milk (10-oz. glass)

BEFORE RETIRING:

Cod Liver Oil Mixture

Suggestions to Overweight People

(1) Eat smaller quantities than you have been eating.
(2) Use only one pat of butter a day.
(3) Drink only 6 oz. of the Common Cold-Preventive Cocktail a day. Do not change the recipe in any way.
(4) For soup, drink only broth and consommé.
(5) Eliminate all coffee and ordinary tea. (I recommend only *herb* teas, to be drunk on an empty stomach. Whenever you feel hungry, drink herb tea—no sugar.)

(6) Raw, unsalted nuts may be eaten, but only several a day (see menus).

(7) The Alexander Vegetable Salad is to be eaten in medium portions.

(8) The Alexander Fruit Salad is to be eaten in small portions.

(9) Drink 6 oz. of milk with lunch and dinner.

(10) No salt is to be used in the diet.

(11) No rich desserts.

(12) No soft drinks.

(13) No frozen juices.

(14) No fried foods. Only broiled.

(15) Don't eat between meals.

Seven Days of Menus for Those Who are Overweight

Monday

BREAKFAST:

Common Cold-Preventive Cocktail
  (6-oz. glass, blended and taken as
  described in Chapter 18)

LUNCH:

Alexander Fruit Salad
  (small portion)
Cottage cheese (1 cup)
Milk (6-oz. glass)

4:00 P.M.

Herb tea (1 cup)

DINNER:

Vegetable broth (1 cup)
Alexander Vegetable Salad (medium portion)
Broiled steak (6 oz.)
Raw carrot sticks (4)
Raw, unsalted Brazil nuts (4)
Milk (6-oz. glass)

10:00 P.M.

Herb tea (1 cup)

Tuesday

BREAKFAST:

Common Cold-Preventive Cocktail
  (6-oz. glass)

LUNCH:

Alexander Vegetable Salad
  (medium portion)
Broiled lean hamburger (6 oz.)
Green celery stalks (2)
Milk (6-oz. glass)

4:00 P.M.

Herb tea (1 cup)

DINNER:

Prime ribs beef (6 oz.)
Baked potato (1 pat butter)
Romaine lettuce and tomato—4 leaves
     and 4 slices
Milk (6-oz. glass)

10:00 P.M.

Herb tea (1 cup)

Wednesday

BREAKFAST:

Common Cold-Preventive Cocktail
     (6-oz. glass)

LUNCH:

Cottage cheese (½ cup)
Fresh peach, sliced
Poached eggs (2)
Canadian bacon (2 slices)
Milk (6-oz. glass)

4:00 P.M.

Herb tea (1 cup)

DINNER:

Alexander Vegetable Salad (medium portion)
Broiled salmon (8 oz.)
Baked potato (1 pat butter)

Raw, unsalted almonds (6)
Milk (6-oz. glass)

10:00 P.M.

Herb tea (1 cup)

Thursday

BREAKFAST:

Common Cold-Preventive Cocktail
(6-oz. glass)

LUNCH:

Sliced hard-boiled egg on romaine lettuce
Whole grain bread (1 slice)
(1 pat butter)
Carrot sticks (4)
Milk (6-oz. glass)

4:00 P.M.

Herb tea (1 cup)

DINNER:

Bouillon (1 cup)
Broiled liver (6 oz.)
Cole slaw (½ cup)
Raw, red onion (1 slice)
Alexander Fruit Salad
(small portion)
Milk (6-oz. glass)

10:00 P.M.

Herb tea (1 cup)

Friday

BREAKFAST:

*Common Cold-Preventive Cocktail
  (6-oz. glass)*

LUNCH:

*Honeydew melon (in season)
  (1 wedge)
Organic hot dogs (2)
  (from health food store)
Baked beans (⅓ cup)
  (no molasses)
Milk (6-oz. glass)*

4:00 P.M.

Herb tea (1 cup)

DINNER:

*Tuna fish salad (medium portion)
Alexander Fruit Salad (small portion)
Pumpkin seeds (1 tablespoon)
Milk (6-oz. glass)*

10:00 P.M.

Herb tea (1 cup)

Saturday

BREAKFAST:

Common Cold-Preventive Cocktail
  (6-oz. glass)

LUNCH:

Consommé (1 cup)
Alexander Vegetable Salad
  (medium portion)
Raw, unsalted Brazil nuts (2)
Milk (6-oz. glass)

4:00 P.M.

Herb tea (1 cup)

DINNER:

Broiled hamburger (8 oz.)
Baked potato (1 pat butter)
Tomato (sliced)
Milk (6-oz. glass)

10:00 P.M.

Herb tea (1 cup)

Sunday

BREAKFAST:

Common Cold-Preventive Cocktail (6-oz. glass)

LUNCH:

Open-faced cheese sandwich
(whole grain bread—1 slice)
Celery stalks (2)
Apple (1)
Milk (6-oz. glass)

4:00 P.M.

Herb tea (1 cup)

DINNER:

Chicken broth (1 cup)
Alexander Vegetable Salad (medium portion)
Broiled chicken (¼ chicken)
Raw, unsalted, assorted nuts mixed with
*   Black Monukka raisins (¼ cup)*
Milk (6-oz. glass)

10:00 P.M.

Herb tea (1 cup)

Cooked Vegetables

I have recommended very few cooked vegetables in the menus because many nutrients are lost in the cooking. However, you will note that in the "Food Substitutions" which follow there are vegetables listed which have to be cooked. To replace the nutrients lost, I recommend the following food supplements, which contain vitamins, minerals and natural enzymes. These can be found in health food stores.

Food Supplements

Bone meal   *Kelp powder*
Brewer's yeast   *Lecithin*
Desiccated liver powder

Food Substitutions

To give more variety in planning your meals, here are foods which can be substituted for those in the menus:

Meats

Chicken   *Roast beef (lean)*
Ham   *Steaks: Sirloin*
Hamburger (lean)   *Porterhouse*
Heart (beef)   *Top round*
Kidneys   *Filet mignon*
Lamb chops (lean)   *T-bone*
Leg of lamb (lean)   *Tongue*
Liver   *Turkey*
Pork (center cut, lean)   *Veal*

Fish

Bluefish   *Crab*
Butterfish   *Flounder*
Clams   *Halibut*
Cod   *Lobster*

Fish (continued)

Mackerel Shrimp
Oysters Swordfish
Pompano Tuna
Salmon Trout
Scallops Whitefish

Vegetables

Alfalfa sprouts Escarole
Asparagus Lettuce (romaine, butter
Beans   and red)
Beets Lima beans
Broccoli Okra
Brussels sprouts Onions
Cabbage Peas
Carrots Peppers
Cauliflower Potatoes
Celery Radishes
Chard Spinach
Corn Squash
Cucumber String beans
Eggplant Tomatoes
Endive

Fresh Fruits

Apples Cantaloupe
Bananas Casaba melon
Blackberries Cherries
Blueberries Crenshaw melon

Fresh Fruit (continued)

Figs

Honeydew melon

Peaches

Pears

Plums

Raspberries

Strawberries

Seeds

Chia

Pumpkin

Sesame

Sunflower

Raw, Unsalted Nuts

Almonds

Brazil nuts

Butternuts

Cashews

Chestnuts

Coconuts

Filberts

Hazel nuts

Peanuts

Pecans

Pinions

Pistachios

Walnuts

Dairy Products

Butter, sweet

Cheeses: American

      Blue

      Cheddar

Cottage

Cream

Swiss

Dairy Products (continued)
Eggs, Fertile and regular
Milk, Raw certified milk, well shaken
Milk, Homogenized, vitamin D
Yogurt, plain
Kefir (liquid yogurt, plain or boysenberry)

Breads

Bran or corn muffins
Brown bread
Chia seed bread
Corn bread
Cracked wheat bread
Graham or rye bread

Pumpernickel
Rye
Soya bread
Sprouted wheat buns
Whole wheat

Natural Organic Honey

All varieties

Herb Teas

All varieties

Part VI
Holidays and
Birthdays

21. The Danger
of Holidays
and Birthday Parties

Holidays

I have found that regardless of temperature, weather and geographical location there is always a high peak of colds during holidays. For example, during Christmas week, in New York the temperature can be freezing, in Hollywood it can be in the 70s, in Australia in the 80s, in New Zealand and in South Africa in the 90s, but, nevertheless, there is a consistent, high peak of colds during Christmas week in all of these places.

Consequently, it became obvious to me that, though the climate differs in these various countries, there must be something in common between all of them. Why should there be such a wave of colds during this holiday week? I analyzed further and discovered that during this holiday people partake

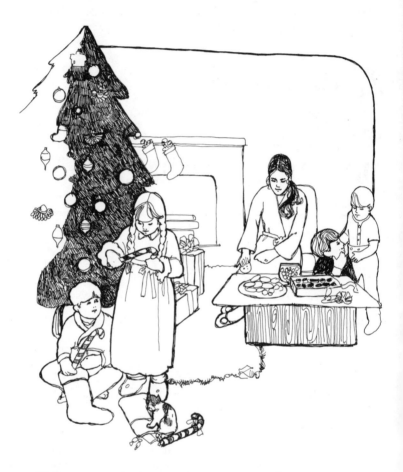

THERE IS ALWAYS A HIGH PEAK OF COLDS DURING CHRISTMAS WEEK
REGARDLESS OF TEMPERATURE, WEATHER AND GEOGRAPHIC LOCATION.
CAUSE—HOLIDAY SWEETS (THROAT IRRITANTS) AND VIRUS.

of *many more sweets*. I had already arrived at my theory that
chocolate and other sticky sweets irritate the mucous lining of
the throat, thereby making it vulnerable to infection by a virus.

I then studied other holidays such as Labor Day, Hallo-
ween, Thanksgiving, Washington's Birthday, St. Valentine's

Day, Easter and Independence Day and found there were also high peaks of colds coincidental with these holidays.

I then found a chart in *The Common Cold,* by Sir Christopher Andrewes, which shows that the higher peaks of colds are in late fall, midwinter and early spring. I checked the calendar and *found these are the holiday periods.* This confirmed my premise. It had already been proven at the Common Cold Research Unit that season, weather and climate do not cause the common cold. Therefore, I concluded that the consumption of sweets as a universal way of celebrating holidays is *the reason* for these high peaks of colds.

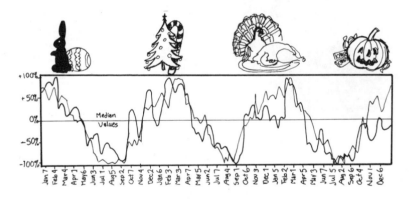

RECORDED HIGH PEAKS OF COLDS ARE COINCIDENT WITH HOLIDAYS, WHEN LARGE QUANTITIES OF SWEET ARE EATEN.

Birthday Parties

This knowledge led me to the realization that, in addition to holidays, there are birthdays which are celebrated with sweets. Young and old carry out the tradition of the frosted birthday cake with candles.

Birthday parties are isolated daily occurrences which can result in cold vulnerability every day of the year if sweets

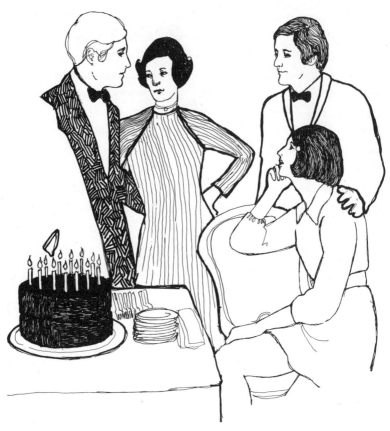

BIRTHDAY CELEBRANTS BECOME COMMON COLD VICTIMS DUE TO
EATING FROSTED CAKE WHEN A COMMON COLD CARRIER IS PRESENT.

are consumed in the presence of someone with a cold. Since
birthdays are not a mass celebration such as holidays, there
are no peaks recorded. However, birthday celebrants are as
much potential cold victims as are holiday celebrants.

Though I have already covered this point, it can bear repeating. Be it a holiday or a birthday, if chocolate or some

other sticky sweet is eaten in the presence of someone with a cold, there is a great likelihood that a cold will result.

I do not mean to discourage people from celebrating holidays and birthdays. They are an integral part of religious, civic and personal tradition. They are observed throughout the world and will continue to be. However, there is a way to enjoy these occasions without danger: *Refrain from chocolate and other sticky sweets!* There are many delicious things which can be eaten such as bowls of unsalted, raw nuts and seeds, a plain, unfrosted cake blazing with candles, natural date and nut cookies, platters of fresh fruit, a punch bowl of fresh, unsweetened fruit juices, assorted sandwiches on whole wheat bread—just to mention a few. (See Chapter 20 for further ideas.)

I assure you, your enjoyment of holidays and birthdays will be complete and no longer dangerous if you carry out my recommendations.

Happy Holidays and Happy Birthday!

Part VII
Questions and
Answers

22. The Mystery of the Common Cold Questions and Answers

Whenever a person catches the common cold, he usually wonders how it happened. In some instances he may think he knows. However, in the main, it is a mystery to him. The following questions and answers will equip the reader with information, clues and the solution to the mystery surrounding the common cold:

QUESTION:

What are the most likely places where the common cold is transmitted and caught?

ANSWER:

Any place where there are common cold carriers present and if chocolate or other sticky sweets are eaten. For ex-

ample, just a few such places are: homes, theatres, schools, public meeting places, conventions, subways and all transportation systems, etc.

QUESTION:

Why do only some people who attend a theatre wake up the following morning with a cold?

ANSWER:

The reason some people wake up with a cold is because they consumed some kind of sticky sweet in the theatre where there were common cold viruses. Those who did not get infected did not eat sweets. Most likely, they ate popcorn, potato chips, hot dogs or sandwiches.

QUESTION:

Is there a high incidence of colds in military barracks?

ANSWER:

Yes, and often they develop into endemic epidemics. The reason is that the G.I. has money in his pocket, time on his hands and a sweet tooth that has to be satisfied.

QUESTION:

Is there a high incidence of colds in penal institutions?

ANSWER:

No. The inmates, as a rule, do not like to eat sweets. Consequently, there are fewer colds.

QUESTION:

Is one more likely to catch a cold at an indoor rather than an outdoor professional sports event?

ANSWER:

Yes. At any gathering indoors the virus can be transmitted more easily. Fortunately, hot dogs, popcorn and beer are more popular than candy at both indoor and outdoor sports events.

QUESTION:

Why are colds more prevalent among school children than adults?

ANSWER:

In school cafeterias, the desserts which most children eat are frequently cake with chocolate frosting, ice cream with chocolate sauce, glazed doughnuts and frosted cupcakes. As a consequence, their throats become irritated from these sticky sweets. If there is someone present who has a cold which is apparent or not, it is almost inevitable that the children who eat the sweets will catch the common cold. An epidemic of the common cold can easily develop in the school because of the sweets. Adults do not eat as many sweets as school children, and, therefore, colds are not as prevalent among them.

QUESTION:

Why do parents and their preschool children catch more colds during the school year than at any other time?

ANSWER:

This is due to the fact that their school children have caught cold as described prior and bring the virus home. If the parents and their preschool children partake of desserts, they, too, are stricken with colds.

QUESTION:

Can parents transmit colds to their children and thereby start an epidemic at school?

ANSWER:

A parent can pick up a virus during the course of the day while consuming sweets and transmit it to his child during dessert. The child then takes it to school, and an epidemic can develop as already described.

QUESTION:

Why do epidemics of the common cold which start in schools spread into the community, while epidemics among new recruits in military barracks remain confined?

ANSWER:

Military recruits make nightly trips to the commissary, where they buy large amounts of candies which they eat when they go back to their barracks. Colds develop as a result of these sweets when there is a common cold carrier present. However, since the new recruits are not permitted to leave the base, they do not spread the virus into the neighboring community. On the other hand, school children consume sweets, catch colds, and because they circulate in the community, they spread the virus.

QUESTION:

Is the "cold season" always coincident with cold weather?

ANSWER:

No. For example, in Australia at Christmas time, the weather is very hot. But even so, there is a short "cold season" during this holiday period.

QUESTION:

What are some typical views on the common cold expressed by doctors?

ANSWER:

A pediatrician: *"The common cold is the most prevalent type of illness in my practice and the most annoying, because it can neither be prevented nor rapidly cured."*
An internist: *"The common cold, in most cases, is not serious. It is rarely fatal."*
A general practitioner: *"Approximately 10 percent of my patients come to me because of the common cold. Science does not yet know the precise cause nor how to cure the common cold. However, it is believed that viruses are at the root of the problem."*
An industrial physician: *"The common cold is a great financial burden. According to National Center for Health*

statistics, colds result in a loss of 46 million work days per year."

QUESTION:

How many common colds are there a year in the United States?

ANSWER:

According to the United States Department of Health, Education and Welfare, "The annual incidence ranges as high as 500 million colds."

QUESTION:

Is there ever a time when a person can eat sweets and not catch cold?

ANSWER:

Yes, providing there is no one present with a cold. However, I want to warn that there can be someone present whose cold is not yet apparent, and this is as dangerous as one with a full-blown cold. Therefore, it is safest to eat sweets only when absolutely alone.

QUESTION:

What percentage of the illnesses that occur in the family in the United States is the common cold?

ANSWER:

According to the Medical Times, *February, 1966, approximately 63.6 percent.*

QUESTION:

What percentage of common cold-like illness is specifically influenza?

ANSWER:

Probably less than 1 percent.

QUESTION:

Why do some infants have very high fevers with their colds?

ANSWER:

There is a virtual absence of antibodies in infants 6 to 9 months of age. Therefore, there is very little resistance. When infection occurs, the body temperature usually rises. Loss of appetite resulting in insufficient fluid intake causes dehydration, which prevents natural cooling from taking place. The infective process itself and the possible dehydration combine to produce a high fever. Whenever there is a high fever, medical attention should be sought, as it can be an indication of complications.

QUESTION:

What percentage of the population in the United States is afflicted with a new cold each week?

ANSWER:

A new cold strikes 13 percent of the entire population every week between the months of September and April. I want to make clear that it is not the same people who are victims each succeeding week. Every week of the year between

*the months of September and April, 13 percent of the popu-
lation is afflicted with a new cold.*

QUESTION:

Within the family, who has more colds—the mother or the
father?

ANSWER:

*The mother. The reason for this is that, in addition to the
fact that she spends more time with the children, she has
more access to sweets and consequently eats them more often.
She also, in many cases, compulsively eats sweets due to the
tensions that occur in raising a family.*

QUESTION:

Who catches more colds—bachelors or married men?

ANSWER:

*Married men. The reason is that many of them are in con-
tact with their children who are frequent victims of the common cold. Though both bachelors and married men eat sweets,
which make them susceptible to the common cold, the married
men catch more colds because of exposure to their children.*

QUESTION:

There are people who claim they have not had a cold in
five years or more. Why is this so?

ANSWER:

The reason is that these people never *eat sweets of any kind, and eat a highly nutritive diet, which helps build resistance.*

QUESTION:

Will a tonsillectomy eliminate future common colds?

ANSWER:

No. The tonsils are not the determining organ in the contraction of a cold. The seat of the problem is the mucous lining of the nose and throat.

QUESTION:

What are antibodies, and what is their function?

ANSWER:

Antibodies are protein molecules, each composed of a chain or chains of hundreds of amino acids. Their function is to fight infection wherever it occurs in the body.

QUESTION:

What is the life-span of a common cold antibody?

ANSWER:

The life-span is between thirty and forty-five days, during which time one is immune to the particular virus which had infected him.

QUESTION:

Does the average medical doctor recognize the importance of nutrition when treating the common cold?

ANSWER:

No. He does not prescribe a nutritive regimen for the illness as does the doctor specializing in nutrition. It is a proven fact that with long-term, consistent, sound nutrition many illnesses can be prevented.

QUESTION:

What might possibly cause an ever-increasing number of common cold viruses?

ANSWER:

One contributing factor may be the prolonged use of adulterated foods. This may cause a change in the biochemical nature of the host cell in the human body. I believe this results in more and more mutations of the viruses.

QUESTION:

Are rhinoviruses just one virus?

ANSWER:

". . . Present members of this group of viruses have been isolated during the past 10 years and have been given various names, such as coryzaviruses and muriviruses. During the past 5 years, particularly due to studies

at the Common Cold Research Unit at Salisbury, England, these agents have been characterized as being similar chemically, physically and biologically and have been collectively designated as rhinoviruses. More than 50 strains—probably subtypes—have been isolated, and there are probably many more: estimates vary from hundreds to even thousands. . . ."[1]

QUESTION:

If a person gets, for example, five different colds in a single season, is he infected by the same virus each time?

ANSWER:

No. Each strain of virus induces firm immunity to itself for a period of thirty to forty-five days. In a volunteer study with a limited number of viruses used, the conclusion was borne out that five colds in one person in a single season were due to five different strains.

QUESTION:

Do 6-month-old infants have antibody immunity to the common cold?

ANSWER:

No. Dr. John H. Dingle, in his article, "The Common Cold and Common-Cold-Like Illnesses" states that there is

---

[1]Dr. John H. Dingle, "The Common Cold and Common Cold-Like Illnesses," *The Medical Times* 94 (February 1966).

". . . virtual absence of antibodies in infants 6 to 9 months of age . . ."

QUESTION:

Why do people catch more colds during the winter months?

ANSWER:

During the winter, once the house or building is heated, the humidity goes down, and the air breathed does not contain enough moisture to keep nose and throat membranes moist. As they dry out, the nose and throat mucous lining is more and more susceptible to cold viruses. It has been established, however, that in the summer, spring and fall, when windows can be opened, the air inside any home or building contains ample moisture, because the earth, grass, leaves and flowers give off moisture all the time. On reasonably cool days, when windows are closed, there is still enough moisture in the air inside, for the house or building continues to hold moisture.

It is the lack of moisture in the air within the home or building, therefore, which is one of the contributing factors for more colds during the winter months. The major cause has been pointed out throughout the book—chocolate and other sticky sweets eaten in the presence of a common cold carrier.

QUESTION:

Do you believe that the common cold starts in the nose?

ANSWER:

There are many who do, but I believe the throat is the

area where a larger percentage of colds begin. I have pointed this out in Chapter 2.

QUESTION:

Why do we suffer from one cold after another?

ANSWER:

The reason why colds may occur repeatedly is that there are many different cold-viruses, and immunity to one does not ensure protection against the others.

QUESTION:

Does dancing or exercise help shorten the time of a cold?

ANSWER:

Mr. J. I. Rodale, the publisher of Why Put Up With Colds, *points out that he had had a severe head cold which settled in his throat. In order to cheer up his two-year-old child, who also had a cold, he started dancing and laughing. As the child reacted with joy, he contorted his body more and more. He then noticed that his voice came back, the soreness disappeared and he could talk with ease. The physical exertion had stimulated his breathing and aided in his recovery.*

QUESTION:

What happens to the continuously moving mucus?

ANSWER:

It moves downward from the upper respiratory tract,

through to the lower respiratory tract, down the esophagus, and finally empties into the stomach. During the course of twenty-four hours, as much as one quart of mucus flows into the stomach.

The minerals and protein in the mucus are digested. Part of the fluid is absorbed. Some part is utilized again by the body, and the waste is eliminated.

QUESTION:

Why is it that some colds last only a day or less?

ANSWER:

Frequently an allergic reaction is mistaken for a cold because the symptoms are similar. For example, one can eat wheat products to which one is allergic and then have all the symptoms of a cold. However, within a short time they disappear. Obviously, therefore, the symptoms were those of an allergy and not a cold.

Also there are times when one feels all the symptoms of a starting cold for a day and then they are gone. His cold was aborted by the natural defenses of the body, which killed the virus.

QUESTION:

What period of time does it take for cold viruses to incubate?

ANSWER:

On the subject of incubation, Sir Christopher Andrewes speaks of six different strains of viruses which were analyzed at the Common Cold Research Unit at Salisbury, England. He states: "Statistical analysis of all the data showed quite clearly that the symptoms produced by these six strains differed significantly, taking them as a whole. It must be 'as a whole' because no one could have drawn conclusions from single volunteers or small numbers. For one thing, the incubation periods were not alike. The mean period from inoculation to beginning of symptoms was 1.4 days for the known rhinovirus DC and for other strains 1.9, 2.2, 2.6, 1.8 days— results in harmony with general experience concerning colds. The GE strain stood apart from the others with a mean incubation period of 3.2 days."

QUESTION:

What happens when a virus infects a cell?

ANSWER:

According to Sir Christopher Andrewes, in his book, The Common Cold:

The protein part of a virus makes specific contact with something on the cell-surface. The cell ingests or takes the virus up within itself. It may ingest the whole virus and break it up inside or, as happens with the bacteriophages or viruses infecting bacteria, the protein coat of the virus may be left outside the cell, only the essential nucleic acid gaining access to the interior. In either event, the protein part of the virus is expendable and plays no further part. The nucleic acid part, however, proceeds to instruct the cellular mechanism in a sinister manner. Suppose it is a rhinovirus infecting a cell lining your nose. The instruction will run thus: 'Stop making the ingredients necessary for making more nose-cells. Henceforth use your chemical laboratory facilities for making more nucleic acid like me.' The intruding virus nucleic acid gives the further instruction: 'And now make a lot of protein of such-and-such composition which I require wherewith to coat myself.' The cell can do nothing but obey and as more new virus particles are thus assembled by the cell's chemical mechanisms they are, at the end of the production line, turned out into the outside of the cell. With many viruses, including probably rhinoviruses, the final effect is to exhaust the cell altogether, so that after a while it dies and disintegrates. The virus set free will infect more of its victim's cells until such time as defence mechanisms have been mobilized. It will also get into the outside world and infect more victims, for one result of the cell-destruction in the course of a cold infection will be inflammation, pouring out of fluid, sneezing and spread of virus. All of it a very conveniently organized affair for the benefit of the rhinoviruses.

QUESTION:

Can viruses be seen?

ANSWER:

Viruses can be seen only with an electron microscope which has great powers of resolution. An electron microscope makes clear a great deal more than an ordinary microscope. It outlines the fine details of virus structure.

QUESTION:

How do chemical pollutants in the air contribute to catching cold?

ANSWER:

Chemical pollutants such as sulphur dioxide both damage the cilia and attack the mucous membrane. (See Chapter 18 regarding cilia and mucous membrane.)

QUESTION:

Can a negative psychological attitude cause a cold?

ANSWER:

It cannot actually cause a cold, but it can affect one's well-being and possibly make one susceptible to the common cold viruses.

Question:

What are the symptoms of a cold?

ANSWER:

The first hint is usually scratchiness in the throat. Within a few hours, your nose gets stuffy, and you have vague feelings of discomfort and illness. Usually you start sneezing, too. Within forty-eight hours, your cold is in full bloom—eyes teary, nose running, voice husky, breathing obstructed, and your senses of taste and smell dulled. You may feel lethargic and achy. It's common to have a moderate headache, especially at the beginning (but a severe one may be a sign of some complication). You may also have some fever, although that's unusual in adults.

QUESTION:

How long does a cold last?

ANSWER:

If there are no complications, a cold will last from several days to two weeks.

QUESTION:

Do the sinuses become involved in colds?

ANSWER:

Some doctors think that involvement of the sinuses occurs in almost all colds. However, we become aware of this only when the infection is severe and particularly when various types of bacteria compound the virus infection, making the cold a serious one. An actual indication of sinus infection is the thick and yellow nasal discharge which is due to pus.

QUESTION:

Can colds lead to serious trouble?

ANSWER:

Yes, at times. This occurs when there is a spread of infection up the Eustachian tube, which can result in middle ear disease. When a person blows his nose too hard, the infected secretions can be pushed into areas where they may do harm. A downward spread may cause laryngitis, tracheitis, bronchitis and even bronchopneumonia.

QUESTION:

When, and under what circumstances, was evidence first found that a virus might be concerned with the common cold?

ANSWER:

Dr. W. Kruse, of the Hygienic Institute of the University of Leipzig, was the first to discover, in 1914, that a virus might be involved. His experimental work consisted of taking the nasal discharge of a cold sufferer and diluting it fifteen times with a saline solution. This was then filtered through a filter which held back all bacteria. With a medicine dropper, he put drops of this up the noses of twelve of his staff. Four of them caught cold after twenty-four to seventy-two hours. Kruse suggested that a virus was concerned. Following this, viral investigation became worldwide.

QUESTION:

Do cats catch cold?

ANSWER:

Yes. Cats very definitely catch cold. A medical authority has stated that cats get bad colds due to several different agents including, possibly, rhinoviruses—but cat rhinoviruses, not human ones.

QUESTION:

Why are some people plagued with colds one winter but not the next?

ANSWER:

It is my belief that these people ate an improper diet during the year they had colds. Then suddenly their diet changed, possibly as a result of learning about sound nutrition. With

the consumption of nutritive foods, they became less vulner-
able to catching cold. This, then, accounts for the winter in
which no colds were caught.

QUESTION:

Why are polar explorers and other isolated groups so
highly susceptible to colds when they make contact with the
rest of the world *after* a long interval?

ANSWER:

While the explorers and isolated groups are away, they are
not in contact with cold viruses. As a consequence no anti-
bodies are built up. Upon their return, therefore, they have
no resistance to any of the many cold viruses circulating in
the community. They are susceptible to these viruses because
they have no reserve of antibodies to fight them.

I should also like to make the point that when they return,
in all likelihood, they partake of rich, sweet desserts. When
these are eaten in the presence of someone with a cold, they
become stricken with colds.

QUESTION:

Do gorillas, orangutans and gibbons catch cold?

ANSWER:

Yes, but there is a lack of evidence as to their cause.

QUESTION:

Can a horse's cold be caught by a human being?

ANSWER:

It was found by Dr. A. Plummer, of the Wellcome Laboratories near London, that when horse virus was inserted up the nose of a human volunteer, he developed a rather severe pharyngitis accompanied by fever. Virus was also recovered from the volunteer's blood. The point was made that, so far as is known, the ordinary rhinoviruses of man do not get into the bloodstream.

QUESTION:

What causes fever blisters?

ANSWER:

Fever blisters are due to the virus of herpes simplex, a virus quite unrelated to those causing colds. Some people carry this virus in a latent state. A cold in some and other stimuli in others, activate this dormant virus, so that these blisters, which soon form scabs and dry up, come along as a complication of a cold.

QUESTION:

Can a cold be caught?

ANSWER:

According to the findings of the Common Cold Research Unit in Salisbury, England, much evidence suggests that a cold can be caught, but it also appears that it is not a very infectious kind of disease.

As already pointed out, colds can be caught if a person

eats chocolate or a sticky sweet in the presence of a cold carrier.

QUESTION:

Are there any statistics and information comparing the common cold in children to that in adults?

ANSWER:

Part of the work at the Common Cold Research Unit in Salisbury, England, involved a study by Dr. T. Sommerville. In making weekly visits to the schools in Chalke Valley, England, where he made records of the occurrence of colds in the children, Dr. Sommerville found that ". . . school children acquired infection outside the household three times as commonly as did adults."

Adults in families containing school children had nearly two-and-a-half times as many colds as did adults in households without children. Infants were the most susceptible but had less opportunity of picking up infection outside the house. The risk that a person in a household with a cold-infection would contract that infection was about one in five. Secondary colds in a house were as likely to pass on to other members as was the first infection to be introduced. This suggests that picking up a cold from a relative is just a matter of chance contact with enough virus in circumstances favorable for the cross-infection to occur. The most significant fiinding from these studies was the important role of children in spreading infection. . . .

QUESTION:

What percentage of cross-infection of common cold occurs from children to adults?

ANSWER:

It has been found to be approximately 10 percent.

QUESTION:

What are some of the possible ways of transmitting common cold infection?

ANSWER:

The following are some of the possible ways:
(1) By coarse droplets reaching a man who is close;
(2) By fine particles remaining suspended long enough to reach a man farther away;
(3) By coarse droplets settling, to be dispersed later as dust.

QUESTION:

Are ultraviolet rays effective in killing airborne viruses?

ANSWER:

Ultraviolet rays have been used in lamps pointing upwards to irradiate the upper layers of air in a room. Circulation of the air should bring germ-bearing particles sooner or later in front of their beams. This has worked very well in laboratory trials but was shown to be far less effective when organisms were protected by the dust or mucus floating along with them. Experiments in England have shown there was some reduction in the number of possibly harmful germs floating in the air, but no reduction at all in the incidence of respiratory infection. One reason for failure of the radiation in such a trial was, of course, that the volunteers only remained in the irradiated room for a part of the day. Possibly the experiment could have worked if all the infection to which the volunteers were exposed was contained in the experimental room. In this way they could not have picked up the infection from other sources.

QUESTION:

Do colds occur in tropical countries?

ANSWER:

Yes, colds do occur in the tropics, but they are less severe and less troublesome than in a temperate climate. For example, in the island of St. John in the Caribbean, colds were reported to be frequent but mild. There were practically no colds from May to October, yet the temperature on that island varies but little.

QUESTION:

Do antihistamine drugs have any curative effect on colds?

ANSWER:

There was a time when antihistamine drugs were used as cold-cures in large quantities. When trials were carried out, however, antihistamines were found to be useless. It is regrettable that years after antihistamines were debunked as cold-cures in scientific journals, they were still being sold in quantity for this purpose.

Nevertheless, it has been found that antihistamines are of benefit against hay fever.

QUESTION:

Does fitness protect one from the common cold?

ANSWER:

According to Sir Thomas Horder, as quoted in The Common Cold *by Sir Christopher Andrewes: "Fitness does not necessarily protect; though with the secondary infections the weakly and tired patient fares worse than the fit."*

However, I have found that good health due to sound nutrition will help build resistance against the common cold.

QUESTION:

When should antibiotics be used?

ANSWER:

According to Wilfred H. Parry, M.D., in an article in Nursing times, *September 16, 1966: "Antibiotics should only be used for complications of colds, such as otitis media, sinusitis, and such lower respiratory tract infections as bronchopneumonia."*

QUESTION:

Can fatigue cause the common cold?

ANSWER:

No. At the University of Illinois, volunteers were kept awake fifty-six hours, but they contracted colds no more readily than well-rested people.

QUESTION:

When nasal discharge thickens and becomes yellowish, what does this indicate?

ANSWER:

This indicates that bacteria, always present in the nose and throat, have taken over the fertile ground prepared by the virus—the raw, inflamed mucous membranes. Researchers have concluded that the viruses prepare the way for an attack by bacteria on throat, nasal and other tissues.

QUESTION:

Has anything been done to cause the cold virus to thrive in a test tube?

ANSWER:

The Salisbury, England researchers had not been able to trap the cold in a test tube where they could study it. Their first problem was to find a diet pleasing to the cold virus, something on which it would thrive in a test tube. For more than a decade the Salisbury workers racked their brains. Bacteria can subsist on almost anything. Viruses, on the other hand, require a diet of living tissue. Researchers in Salisbury, as a result of work done at Harvard University, tried to grow *the cold virus with kidney tissue from monkeys, but had no luck. They then tried it with human kidney cells. The virus appeared to grow on the human kidney cells, but growth was feeble.*

Then a laboratory accident occurred. As nourishment in the laboratory, the kidney cells had been given a diet of a standard culture medium called 199, which was a mixture of vitamins, minerals, amino acids and bicarbonate of soda. Suddenly, the cold virus began to grow with enthusiasm never observed before. It even left behind clear, microscopic evidence of having attacked and damaged the kidney cells. Here was the beginning of the first laboratory test for cold virus. After checking, researchers found that, through an error, the 199 culture contained only half the bicarbonate of soda called for. This lessened-alkalinity was precisely what the cold virus wanted.

Out of this work came the realization that the first step in production of a protective vaccine is to grow virus or bacteria in a laboratory, readily and in quantity. The virus is then killed or weakened to make it safe for use.

QUESTION:

What percentage of the population in the United States catches colds in the winter months as compared to the percentage in the summer months?

ANSWER:

From The American Journal of Nurses, *December, 1963, in an article by Dr. Lewis B. Lefkowitz, Jr., 15 percent of the entire population has some sort of respiratory infection during*

*the two summer quarters; and 50 percent of the entire popu-
lation has some sort of respiratory infection during the two
winter quarters.*

QUESTION:

Are there any drugs that can kill viruses?

ANSWER:

*A cold is an infection with a virus—a type of germ that
can't be knocked out even by wonder drugs. In fact the first
drugs that actually kill viruses are just now being developed
and tested. Only three have emerged, and those in the last
ten years. And it is this discovery— that such antiviral agents
do exist—that is an important part of the cold-cure rush.*

QUESTION:

Are there any cold remedies that can be harmful?

ANSWER:

*Large quantities of liquids are frequently recommended,
but their value is open to question. . . . Nose drops and
inhalers shrink the membrane of the nose and so give
temporary relief of stuffiness and nasal congestion. Unfortunately, use of these drugs frequently results in more
swelling than was present before. . . . Most preparations
stop the action of and often actually destroy the cilia. . . .*

Studies have shown that there is no justification for the use of antihistamine drugs, sulfonamides, or antibiotics. Some people have undesirable reactions to these drugs. Also if these drugs are used for colds, strains of germs that are resistant to them may develop; and the drugs become valueless for the treatment of severe infections. . . .[1]

In discussing cold remedies with a physician in Los Angeles, I learned that one of the fallacies in treating the common cold is that which urges the consumption of cold drinks, because they lower the tissue temperature, making a favorable atmosphere for germs. The physician pointed out that mucus is the best protection against the common cold. He is cautious about prescribing antihistamines. He will do so only if the nose is running; but he will not do so for a sore throat. He further said that when you dry up the mucus, you change the thickness of the viscosity of the mucus. He emphasized the fact that mucus is important because it is the protecting blanket of the mucous membrane. Not only are antihistamines bad for the mucus but so is heating. If one dries out the mucus, he gets microscopic fissures or ruptures deep in the mucous lining, thus making one more vulnerable to the germs.

QUESTION:

What are the statistics on colds in the United States?

---

[1]*Encyclopaedia Britannica,* 1969 edition, vol. 6 (published by Encyclopaedia Britannica, Inc.) pp. 42 and 43.

ANSWER:

Surveys indicate that approximately 75 percent of the people of the United States have at least one cold each year and 25 percent have four or more.

QUESTION:

Why don't nonrecruit military populations have the same common cold epidemic patterns as new recruits?

ANSWER:

The life of commissioned and noncommissioned officers differs from that of the new recruits. Whereas recruits spend a lot of their leisure time in the commissary, where they eat large quantities of sweets, the officers prefer taverns, sports, theatre and other diversions to sweets. Consequently, the officers do not become common cold victims as frequently. Therefore, they do not have the same common cold epidemic patterns as new recruits.

QUESTION:

Is there a vaccine which will give immunity to the common cold?

ANSWER:

No, because there are too many common cold viruses. Since a vaccine is made from only one virus, obviously it will not immunize one against all the existing viruses.

QUESTION:

Does a sturdy, healthy body produce a high level of natural immunity to the common cold?

ANSWER:

Yes. One in good health does not catch cold easily.

QUESTION:

Is coughing always a harmful symptom?

ANSWER:

Coughing at times can be helpful, because it aids in the preservation of the physical integrity of the lungs.

QUESTION:

What are the symptoms of influenza?

ANSWER:

The overall symptoms are shivery chilliness, headache, body aching, extreme fatigue, temperature over 101° in adults and 104° and up in children. The older one is, the more severe the symptoms. The fever lasts about three days, after which the symptoms begin to lessen.

QUESTION:

What is pneumonia?

ANSWER:

Pneumonia is a severe inflammation of either one or both lungs, caused by either a virus or bacteria. The most common type of pneumonia is caused by pneumococcus bacteria.

QUESTION:

Is the use of drugs containing ephedrine advisable?

ANSWER:

Dr. Noah D. Fabricant, in his book, The Dangerous Cold, *points out that an important argument against overuse of these is they affect the motion of the nasal cilia. "The vasoconstrictor substances have absolutely no curative effects on the cold itself, since they only relieve one of its mechanical symptoms, nasal congestion, and do so only temporarily. . . ."*

QUESTION:

Are there any over-the-counter cures for the common cold?

ANSWER:

No. But some of these will alleviate a headache, soothe a sore throat and reduce a moderate fever.

QUESTION:

What is the proper way to blow the nose?

ANSWER:

Do not blow hard. Instead, blow softly and repeatedly. Blow with both nostrils wide open. Avoid shutting off one nostril, as it will cause pressure on the other one. This action forces mucus into the Eustachian tube, which can cause a middle ear infection.

QUESTION:

Does humidification help one with a bad cold?

ANSWER:

Yes. When used, the cilia which have been immobilized by the dryness will function again and possibly defeat the cold germs by themselves.

QUESTION:

Is it beneficial to drink liquids when one has a cold?

ANSWER:

Yes, if the right kind of liquids are drunk. I recommend hot herb teas, since these have a healing effect on the body, and also limited amounts of fresh orange juice at room temperature. Do not drink frozen or canned juices or soft drinks. It is preferable to drink hot liquids rather than cold, since the heat is soothing and prevents internal thermal shock.

QUESTION:

What do you think of aspirin?

ANSWER:

Aspirin is a popular medication and if used according to directions, has almost no side effects. It makes the common cold victim more comfortable. When there is a moderate fever, aspirin reduces it, and allays aches and pains. However, it is not a cure. Unfortunately, it can relieve symptoms so much that the common cold victim goes out before he should, which can result in a return of the symptoms with worsening infection.

QUESTION:

Is alkalinization advisable in the treatment of a common cold?

ANSWER:

No. People were wrong when they used large quantities of baking soda in water as a means of counteracting acidity which was believed to be one of the reasons for a cold. There is no scientific proof that any alkaline substance is of value in treating a cold. Experiments were conducted at the University of Minnesota on the effects of baking soda on colds, using much larger doses than are available in commercial preparations, and it was found that the therapeutic results were entirely negative.

QUESTION:

Are nose drops of value in treating nasal colds?

ANSWER:

Yes, but only if prescribed by a doctor. The drops offer temporary relief. They are of value because they make it possible for air to reach the upper part of the nose, thus freeing the cilia to remove bacteria from the mucous membrane. The vasoconstrictors in the nasal medication reduce the swelling, thereby opening the way for the natural defenses of the body to operate effectively. Also, the use of nose drops in many cases is sufficient to make the cold symptoms disappear.

QUESTION:

Do mentholated cigarets bring relief from symptoms of a cold?

ANSWER:

They may cool the nostrils temporarily, but they very definitely irritate the nose and throat tissues, and should be avoided as should all kinds of tobacco.

QUESTION:

Will a laxative or cathartic aid in elimination of the infection of a cold?

ANSWER:

No. They should be used only for constipation. They will not purge a cold.

QUESTION:

Do gargles help cure a cold?

ANSWER:

There is divided opinion on this. Some doctors prescribe

*gargling with hot salt water, whereas other doctors say it is
of no value because it cannot reach the germs which are deep
in the throat tissues.*

QUESTION:

What are viruses immune to?

ANSWER:

*They are immune to practically any substance other than
antibodies within the body.*

QUESTION:

What occurs when vitamin C is taken to make it such an
excellent form of therapy?

ANSWER:

*F. R. Klenner, M.D., of Reidville, N. C., has used vitamin
C successfully in the treatment of many serious diseases. In a
paper which he presented before the Fifty-second Annual
Meeting of the Tri-State Medical Association of the Carolinas
and Virginia, February 19 and 20, 1951, he describes his
point of view. He compares the action of vitamin C with that
of antibiotics. "It has been reported," he says, "that one of
the mold-derived drugs (antibiotics) is a super-vitamin." Dr.
Klenner believes that it is the capacity of the vitamin as an
aid to oxidation that makes it valuable against germs. It
seems to unite with the toxin of virus and helps to destroy it.*

QUESTION:

Are there any sticky sweets which will not irritate the

throat lining and cause the common cold?

ANSWER:

Yes. All sticky sweets which have been left in their natural state and have not been refined or processed. For example, natural organic honey is such a sweet. These will not cause the common cold.

QUESTION:

Why will some people get "cold symptoms" from natural sweets?

ANSWER:

Those people are allergic to natural sweets. Do not confuse an allergy with the common cold even though their symptoms are similar.

QUESTION:

Does yogurt become cold-causing when it is mixed with artificial, sticky sweet, fruit flavoring?

ANSWER:

Very definitely yes. This flavoring is an irritant and can cause the common cold if eaten in the presence of a common cold victim. I want to make clear that this does not apply to plain yogurt which is nutritious.

QUESTION:

Is vitamin C perishable?

ANSWER:

Yes, it is the most perishable vitamin there is. It is lost when foods are cooked. It seeps away into the water when foods are soaked.

QUESTION:

Can a person suffer from the lack of only one vitamin?

ANSWER:

Single deficiencies seldom occur naturally. In terms of human nutrition, a person who suffers from a lack of one B vitamin is certain to lack the others too, for they occur mostly in the same foods, and they react with one another in the body. Someone who lacks vitamin B will probably lack vitamin C as well. If a person does not get enough vitamin A in his food, he almost certainly will not get enough of the other fat soluble vitamins—D and E—for they occur in many of the same foods.

QUESTION:

What do some virologists and biochemists hope to achieve with regard to the common cold?

ANSWER:

They hope that some day they may be able to "immunize" the nucleic acid in the cells of normal living bodies so that the virus invasion will be negated, and thereby wipe out much illness.

Part VIII
People

23. Appeal to People in the Public Eye

People who are in the public eye or work with the public cannot afford to catch a cold. Though they may think they can carry on their work in spite of a cold, they cannot function effectively. For example:

Politics

Supposing a candidate for the presidency of the United States, at the most crucial part of his campaign, should catch a cold. What might the consequences be? Let us say, according to the polls, his opponent is running very close behind. Last-minute speeches in person and on television can help determine the outcome of the election. Apart from his platform, the candidate's voice is a most important requisite. If, because of a cold, he practically loses his voice but nevertheless attempts to speak, there will not be sufficient force to carry through his convictions and inspire confidence in him. In the event he appoints someone to read his speech for him, it will obviously lose its impact.

A presidential candidate has the enormous responsibility to appear before the public as scheduled and to be in good health and good voice. A cold may seem inconsequential, but it can mean the difference between winning the election or losing it, and thereby can affect the fate of the world.

Sports Events

Supposing the key quarterback on a major, professional football team should catch cold the day of the Super Bowl game being played for the World Championship. What are the consequences? His energy is low. His breathing is impaired. His eyes water and his nose runs. His body aches. The teams are two points apart with just ten seconds to play. The quarterback is the star of the team and has made a valiant attempt to keep going. However, the coach sees the shape he is in. A decision has to be made, whether to risk keeping him in for the final play or sending in a substitute quarterback.

Such an important member of the team has the responsibility to be in good shape. His cold can mean the difference between his team's winning the national championship and a bonus of a higher percentage of gate receipts, or losing and a smaller percentage of gate receipts.

Theatre Performances

Supposing the star of a Broadway play should catch a cold on opening night. What occurs? She has a hacking cough, hoarse voice and a low level of energy. Her part in the play calls for great variation of voice, much vitality and beauty. The curtain is about to go up. The director sees her red eyes, red nose, and hears the crack in her voice. He has to decide whether to let her go on and risk the producers' quarter-million dollars, the playwright's future and the fate of the play, or to put on her understudy—also very risky.

The star of the play has the responsibility to appear and perform with her full potential. Her cold can mean the difference between good reviews and a long run, or a panning and close of the play.

Opera

Supposing a new tenor who is making his debut singing Rodolfo in La Bohème at the La Scala in Italy is struck with a cold. What happens? His throat is raw and inflamed. His voice is raspy and uncontrolled. The audience is eager to hear this new talent. The critics are waiting. The entire cast is behind him. The director comes in to wish him well and hears his grating voice express anxiety. What to do? Will he be able to sing? Can the risk be taken?

When so much has been invested in the new tenor, he has the responsibility to the producers, the company, the audience and to his career to stay well. His cold can mean the difference between success or failure.

Ballet

Supposing a Russian prima ballerina should catch cold just before she is to appear at a command performance at Covent Garden in London, England. What happens? She sneezes. Her chest is congested. Her wind is impaired. Her body aches. Her legs are tense. The Queen and royal family sit in their box awaiting her entrance. The prima ballerina has difficulty backstage limbering up. Everyone in the company is sympathetic and encouraging. She cries out she cannot dance. The cold has taken its toll on her body.

When so much is at stake, the prima ballerina has the responsibility to dance. Her cold can mean disappointment to the Queen, the royal family, the audience, and a sense of failure for herself.

Other Types of Work

There are countless men and women who may not be in the "star" realm but who, nevertheless, do important work dealing with the public. They, too, have the responsibility to appear according to schedule, be it at a religious gathering, school function, lecture, or sales meeting—just to mention a few.

Should they be struck with a cold, the result could be either spiritual denial to the congregation, inconvenience, disappointment, refunds, disruption of plans or substantial monetary loss.

My Appeal

Since this book explains how the common cold is caught, how to avoid it, how to stay well and as a consequence be able to perform one's work, I appeal to all people to pay heed to what causes the common cold, to refrain from the dangerous beverages and foods mentioned herein, and to follow the nutritional regimen recommended in this book. The results will be greatly desired good health—free of colds— and the ability to function on all fronts.

Index